COUNT
YOUR
CALORIES

THE PAPERBACK

COUNT YOUR CALORIES

Editor
Dr Amanda Roberts

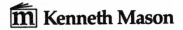 Kenneth Mason

Published by Kenneth Mason
Dudley House, 12 North Street, Emsworth, Hants PO10 7DQ
0243 377977

Adapted from The Composition of foods (4th Edition), which is Crown copyright,
with the permission of the Controller of Her Majesty's Stationery Office.

© Dr Amanda Roberts, introduction, 1990, 1992
© Kenneth Mason Publications Ltd, tables, 1990, 1992

British Library Cataloguing in Publication Data
Roberts, Amanda
    The Paperback count your calories.
    1. Food. Calorific values
    I. Title
    641.1'042

ISBN 0-85937-350-9

Contents

Section 2 continued

Section 3 - Alcohol listings

INTRODUCTION

What are calories and kilojoules?
A calorie is a measure of energy. Kilojoules are the metric equivalent and one calorie is equal to 4.184 kilojoules.

The calorie value of foods in the following tables shows how much energy a hundred grammes or one ounce of that food provides after you have eaten it.

Every day we use a large number of calories even if we just lie around in bed. We need calories to keep our heart beating, for breathing, to maintain our body temperature and for our brain to function. Physical work requires many more calories and any kind of exercise whether for work, pleasure or to lose weight will increase our calorie needs. Any calories we eat which are not used will be stored by our bodies. Extra calories are stored as fat.

So we gain fat when our calorie intake is greater than our calorie needs. We lose fat when we eat slightly less calories than we need.

Why we should count calories
Calorie controlled diets have long been popular as a way of reducing weight. As a form of dieting it is accessible to everyone and does not involve great expense or even great changes in diet.

Nearly forty percent of the population of Great Britain is overweight. This is mainly because they eat too much; their calorie intake is too high. Many overweight people could balance their high calorie intake by exercising more but most have neither the time nor inclination to do so. The more overweight you are the less you feel like exercising. Counting calories to help reduce weight can be the first stage in feeling healthier and more energetic. Being over-weight is not only uncomfortable and bad for morale but also bad for our health by putting increased strain on our hearts and joints.

If our intake of calories is less than the amount we require each day our bodies will use stored energy. Most of our stored energy exists as fat. By eating slightly less than our required calorie intake we will lose fat. Our bodies need calories to mobilise and convert these fat stores to energy. If we reduce our intake too much we have insufficient calories to mobilise stores and we end up listless and irritable without the fat loss desired.

When to count calories
It is important to know what we are eating all the time. After dieting it is important to maintain the correct weight. Having a rough idea about calories and food values can prevent business lunches or special dinners becoming calorie disasters. A little knowledge helps prevent choosing the dish with the highest calories in every course, and helps monitor our daily intake.

So we should count our calories all the time. This does not mean painstakingly weighing all our food or calculating exact values before we eat anything. It means reading through and comparing food values, remembering the values of our preferred foods and snacks and taking care to avoid certain foods while eating others more freely.

How to count your calories
Before starting on a calorie controlled diet you will need to assess your current calorie intake. Use the tables to calculate your intake on an average weekday with an evening meal at home and an average weekend day or holiday with a meal out. Add the total for both days and halve it to give an average figure. To be more accurate assess your daily intake for a whole week and divide by seven. Remember almost everyone underestimates their intake.

There is considerable variation in the amount of food or calories required by individual people, therefore diets like '1000 calories a day' are unhelpful and sometimes dangerous.   Never set your goal below 1000 calories a day without medical supervision.

Has your weight increased over the past few months or stayed the same? If it is constant reduce your intake initially by 250 calories daily.   If you have gained weight reduce your daily intake by 500 calories.   This applies even if your intake is very high.   Reducing by a large amount suddenly is hard to adjust to and therefore less likely to be successful.

Calorie requirements depend on age, sex and occupation as well as exercise and general health.   From our mid twenties our calorie requirements decrease but our intake, if anything, increases - you see the origins of 'middle age spread'.

The average 30 year old man uses between 2000 to 3000 calories a day while the average 30 year old woman uses between 1450 to 2250 calories.   Yet if you imagine the different amounts of energy used by a secretary sitting typing all day and a housewife running a house and chasing around after small children you can see how unhelpful these average figures can be.   Anyone starting a calorie controlled diet must set their own goal based on their current levels of intake.

A calorie controlled diet involves careful planning and care to ensure that your calorie intake comes from a variety of foods and includes adequate carbohydrates, fat, fibre and protein.

Recommended weights for health

Over the page is a chart with recommended weights for different heights of men and women once they have reached their eighteenth birthday. As you will see there is a considerable range of acceptable weight for each height just as

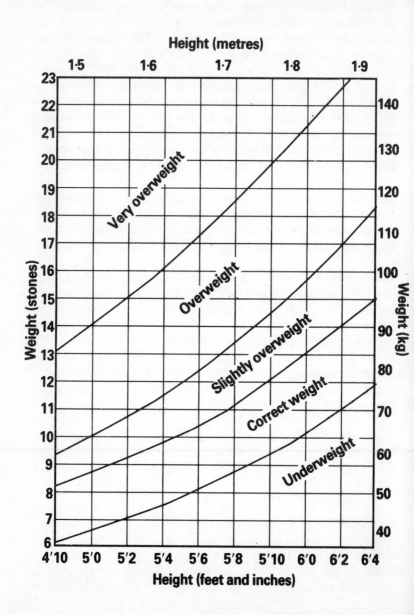

there is huge variation in the amount of calories different people require so there is an equally large variation in individual builds: some people have wide shoulders and hips, some short bodies and long legs... The ratio of muscle to fat in your body affects your weight. A man who 'works out' regularly and plays a lot of sport may well weigh more than a man of the same height who is fatter and takes no exercise. As muscle weighs more than fat a thinner person does not necessarily weigh less. To find an ideal weight for each individual we need to consider many more factors than mere height. But if you are in the upper part of the weight band for your height and know you have a slight rather than a stocky build you should probably lose some surplus pounds. If you are outside the band in the overweight section you should definitely lose weight. If in the underweight section you should aim to put on weight by building up your muscles and eating a healthy high calorie diet.

Never aim to weigh less than the lowest recommended weight for your height even if you are unhappy with your shape or how you look. Instead seek professional advice at a gym and start an exercise programme, and take medical advice on how to achieve your desired shape.

Surplus weight can lead to serious medical problems: if you are worried on this score always seek medical advice.

Balancing the source of our calories & why we need a variety of foods

The food we eat should contain a mixture of protein, carbohydrate, fat, vitamins and minerals. No single food can supply all of these. We need therefore a balanced diet - and variety in our foods.

Our daily calorie intake comes from fats, carbohydrates and proteins. Vitamins and minerals are essential for proper functioning of our bodies and for absorption and utilisation of different nutrients. We need the B vitamins to metabolise

fats, carbohydrates and proteins; vitamin C to absorb iron
and vitamin D to utilise calcium. We need fibre, an indigestible carbohydrate with no calorie value, to keep our
bowels regular and our digestive system healthy. Often
various nutrients have to be eaten at the same time which is
why meals of more than one foodstuff are necessary.

Some fat is essential in our diet to supply fat-soluble vitamins and essential fatty acids which our bodies cannot
synthesise. Normally no more than a quarter of our daily
calories should come from fat. When dieting it is advisable
to have a lower fat intake than this as fat has the highest
calorie quota before satisfying pangs of hunger.

Our protein intake should be 11% of our daily calorie count
but protein requirement is a complex problem. We need a
variety of proteins in our diet to provide the eight essential
amino acids our bodies cannot make and for the amino acids
made in our bodies we need the precursors in correct
proportions for the amino acids which are made in our
bodies.

The calories provided by carbohydrates are interchange-
able with those from fats but it is recommended that carbohydrates provide between 50% and 70% of our calories.
Varying our source of calories as well as our sources of fats,
carbohydrates and proteins should supply all essential
vitamins and minerals. Nonetheless while on a low calorie
diet it is advisable to take a multivitamin supplement once
a day.

Protein
The main building block of our bodies, protein, promotes
tissue growth and repair. Even when we have reached our
optimum height our bodies constantly renew and repair
tissues. Skin, muscles, bones, nerves and blood all depend
on the amino acids found in dietary protein. There are 22
amino acids which make up proteins in various

combinations.   As eight of these amino acids cannot be synthesised by our bodies they must be supplied by our diet.

Most of us think first of red meat as the prime source of protein but beware: it contains a lot of hidden fat. Fish, poultry and white meat are healthier sources with lower calorific values.

Milk, eggs and cheese are high protein foods.   Good vegetable sources include cereals, nuts, pulses (beans & lentils) and wholemeal bread.   Vegetable proteins can easily provide us with our daily requirements so we need not depend on meat. By cutting down or even cutting out meat from our diets we benefit from a lower fat intake.

Carbohydrates

These supply energy for the body's immediate use including digesting and using other nutrients such as fat and protein.   Stores of carbohydrates in the body are only enough to supply energy for a day or less. These stocks are constantly replenished from body fat which may last for months.   A low calorie diet works by using up your carbohydrate reserve and by breaking down body fats which replenish it.

Apart from supplying energy quickly carbohydrates also play a vital role in the functioning of the liver and brain, and in heart and muscle contraction.

There are three groups of carbohydrates: sugar, starch and fibre.

The simplest carbohydrates are the sugars. These include fructose – found in fruits; lactose – found in milk; and glucose and sucrose. Sucrose usually appears in our diets as white or brown refined sugar, is unnecessary and contributes little by way of nutrition. By cutting down on sucrose intake you will be helped to lose weight without missing any essential nutrients.

Starches, broken down to glucose by the body, are found in most plant foods such as cereals, rice, vegetables and legumes. Starchy foods such as bread and potatoes provide carbohydrate combined with protein, minerals and vitamins as well as fibre.

Fibre is the indigestible carbohydrate part of plants. In the last 25 years we have become far more aware of the importance of a high fibre content in our diet and its relation to health. Communities with a high fibre diet have a lower incidence of diseases of the bowel including cancer.

Fibre absorbs moisture as it passes through the bowel making bowel actions softer, bulkier and more regular. If you increase your fibre intake match it with a corresponding amount of extra fluid.

The best sources of dietary fibre are whole grain cereals, fruits, pulses such as beans and lentils, bran and unpeeled potatoes.

Fats
Like carbohydrates, fats fall into three main groups: saturated, polyunsaturated and monounsaturated. Their main dietary role is as a source of energy providing more than twice as many calories per gramme than either protein or carbohydrate.

Western diets tend to contain an unhealthy amount of fat. In the USA more than 40 per cent of their total calories often comes from fat, whereas it supplies only 8-10 per cent in Japan. Our fat intake in the UK is close to the Americans: it should be halved.

Saturated fats such as butter, many margarines, cheese and lard are usually solid at room temperature. Animal fats contain more saturated fats than their vegetable equivalents. Coconut oil is unusual in being a saturated vegetable fat.

Polyunsaturated and monounsaturated fats are found mainly in vegetable oils, such as groundnut , sunflower, vegetable and olive oils. They are liquid at room temperature.

Most fats are a mixture of these three, saturated, polyunsaturated and monounsaturated.   The number of calories present depends on the total fat content rather than its type. Research into general health and heart disease has shown both that a diet low in saturated fats is healthier and that unsaturated fats such as are found in fish oils may help prevent heart disease.

Cholesterol is a product of fat metabolism as well as being present in certain foods. It has gained a bad name because high blood cholesterol so often accompanies heart disease. Cholesterol is a vital raw material for making certain body hormones and bile salts: only when levels of cholesterol in the blood are too high is it considered unhealthy.

Vitamins

Vitamin C
This vitamin is necessary to maintain a healthy skin and is important in the formation of collagen in the body to help healing. Vitamin C deficiency is not unknown in western society and causes a disease called scurvy where skin tissue breaks down. The vitamin is also involved in the formation of blood, hormone production and assists the absorption of iron into the body.

As a water soluble vitamin it cannot be stored in the body, therefore a daily intake is necessary, ideally with some at each meal.

A great deal of this vitamin can be lost during cooking and preserving. It is important therefore not to cook food longer than necessary. Vegetables cooked until they are soggy will have lost most of this vitamin and boiled milk about 50% of its original vitamin C content.

Vitamin C is found mainly in fruit and vegetables, both fresh and frozen. Particularly good sources are citrus fruits such as oranges and grapefruit, kiwi fruit, strawberries and potatoes eaten with their skins.

Vitamin B
These are also water soluble and are not significantly stored in the body. There are many different B vitamins with different functions but they are grouped together as they are found in a great variety of foods and depend on each other to function.

They are important in the metabolism of fats, carbohydrates and proteins and in the manufacture of haemoglobin, RNA and DNA and the normal functioning of the nervous system. Like vitamin C they can be destroyed by over cooking and sometimes even by low heat or sunlight. Milk left standing in the sun loses B vitamins rapidly.

The five main B vitamins are
1 Vitamin B_1 or Thiamine which is important in the metabolism of food to release energy. It is found in a variety of foods including whole grain cereals and breads, pork, legumes and sweetcorn, figs and prunes.

2 Vitamin B_2 or Riboflavin has a function similar to Vitamin B_1 and is found in many foods including milk and dairy products, white meat, liver, cereals, nuts, mushrooms and broccoli as well as eggs.

3 Vitamin B_3 or Nicotinic acid has the same function as B_1 and B_2. Good sources of this vitamin include meat espe-

cially liver, peanut butter, whole grain cereals, avocado and potatoes.

4 Vitamin B_6 or Pyridoxine as well as being necessary for food metabolism is essential for the formation of adequate haemoglobin in the blood. Good sources are meat, fish, milk, egg yolks, bananas, avocados, carrots and pineapple.

5 Folic acid is important in the formation of RNA and DNA in the nuclei of all our cells and becomes increasingly important during pregnancy. It is found in all foods except fats and sugar, but particularly in meat, liver, green leafy vegetables, nuts and fruits especially oranges and bananas.

6 Vitamin B_{12} is important in haemoglobin formation too but is found only in meat, eggs and dairy produce. Vitamin B_{12} is not found in plant foods so strict vegetarians need an external supplement.

All the B vitamins apart from Vitamin B_{12} are found in high concentrations in nutritional yeast or brewers yeast which is often supplemented with B_{12} to provide an adequate supply of the whole group.

Fat soluble vitamins
Vitamin D
Vitamin D is necessary for maintenance and formation of healthy bone. It is stored in our livers and kidneys.

The main source of vitamin D is sunlight. When our skins are exposed to it we ensure a good supply of the vitamin. It is provided in our diet by oily fish, eggs, liver and kidneys. Too much in the diet is toxic and can be dangerous. Our bodies control the amount of vitamin D made in the skin and we cannot acquire too much from sunlight alone.

Vitamin A
This vitamin helps our bodies fight infections and strengthens

the skin and membranes in our bodies. It is vital to good eyesight and in the synthesis of RNA in cell nuclei.

There are two types of Vitamin A: preformed or retinol which is found in animal fats and is toxic if too much is eaten. The second type is carotene found in green and yellow vegetables and is not toxic. Carotene is best absorbed if these vegetables are cooked or mashed up. Vitamin A is stored in our livers.

Good food sources include full fat milk, dairy products, egg yolks, liver and oily fish. Vegetable sources include dark leaves of leafy vegetables and carrots.

Vitamin E
Many claims about the powers and functions of this vitamin have been made but few proven or accepted. Found in all our cell membranes it helps healing and slows ageing of the skin. It also assists our bodies to use other vitamins. We get rid of excess Vitamin E quickly and toxicity is rare. Good dietary sources include vegetable oils, nuts and seeds, avocados, whole cereals, oily fish and spinach.

Vitamin K
Is essential to make prothrombin, a part of our system of blood clotting. It is found in plant foods and is also made by bacteria living in the human gut. Our main dietary sources are leafy green vegetables, yoghurt, egg yolks and polyunsaturated oils.

As you can see it is the water soluble vitamins which are not stored in our bodies and which we need to eat every day especially when dieting. The fat soluble vitamins are stored in the body so daily intake is less essential. Vitamins A and D are toxic if too much is taken so causing serious health problems. Poisoning from these vitamins is not unheard of in people taking excessive cod or halibut liver oil supplements. Vitamins contain no calories but are an essential part of our diet.

Minerals

These are essential nutrients for growth, maintenance and proper functioning of our bodies. They contain no calories.

Calcium

This is the main mineral found in our bodies, particularly in our bones and teeth. Once we stop growing our skeletons are still being constantly replaced and repaired for which we need a regular supply of this mineral. Calcium is also necessary for blood-clotting and for nerve and muscle function including the continuous beating of heart muscle.

Our prime dietary source is dairy products with milk being the most important. Skimmed milk has a calcium content similar to ordinary milk though it has fewer calories. Other sources are fish, especially those with edible bones like tinned sardines, dark green vegetables, potatoes, dried figs, nuts, hard (chalky) water and bread, as calcium is often added to the flour.

We need vitamin D to absorb calcium.

Magnesium

Is also necessary for bone formation and essential for the absorption of other minerals and vitamins. Magnesium is found in meat, whole grain cereals, green vegetables and nuts.

Iodine

This mineral is essential for the correct functioning of the thyroid gland. The iodine content of fruit and vegetables depends on the make-up of the soil in which they are grown. In certain areas the soil and water are iodine depleted so supplements are sometimes needed. Iodine is also found in fish, shellfish, fish oil and table salt (to which it has been added).

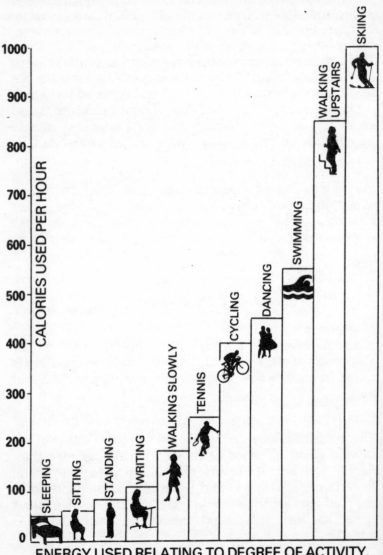

ENERGY USED RELATING TO DEGREE OF ACTIVITY.
THE VALUE WILL VARY ACCORDING TO INDIVIDUAL EXERTION.

Zinc
The importance of this mineral is becoming increasingly recognised. It is necessary in many bodily reactions and in the formation of DNA and RNA as well as participating in the healing process. Good sources include meat and dairy products, nuts and lentils, cocoa, sweetcorn and fresh mango.

Sodium
Most sodium is added to our food as salt (sodium chloride). It is impossible *not* to get adequate sodium in our diet; indeed most of us eat far more salt than we need. To eat less salt avoid buying preprepared or ready cooked foods, add less and less salt to food when cooking and gradually your taste will adapt. Low sodium diets are still recommended for those with high blood pressure, even though, researchers have not proved there is a relationship between the two.

Iron
Is essential for the formation of haemoglobin in our red blood cells. Iron is not well absorbed from the gut without an adequate intake of vitamin C. Good sources of iron include red meat, liver and kidney, egg yolks, shrimps and fish. Vegetarians obtain adequate iron from beans, lentils and cereals. Reasonable amounts of iron are also found in apricots and peaches, chocolate, spinach and watercress.

Exercising on a calorie controlled diet
Most of us should exercise more than we do both for fitness and physical shape. Undertaking a heavy new exercise programme or aerobics class at the same time as commencing a low calorie diet is dangerous. Your calorie need will increase dramatically as you reduce your intake. Expect therefore to feel tired and irritable as well as hungry!

The best exercises on a calorie-controlled diet are brisk walking, swimming or cycling. These three forms of exercise are ideal for getting and staying fit without stress to joints and muscles. Brisk walking is probably as beneficial as jogging. Moderate exercise three times a week is better than strenuous exercise once a week. There is no need to go bright red, sweaty and exhausted in order to lose and keep down your weight. Moderate regular exercise is the answer.

Start exercising a couple of weeks *before* or *after* you go onto your calorie-controlled diet and, if necessary, remember to increase your calorie allowance accordingly. You may well need another 500-750 calories per day if you start swimming for an hour three times a week. These calories will help you exercise more efficiently yet still allow calories from your stores of fat to be used up.

Menus

Menu 1	calories per serving	*Menu 2*	calories per serving
Whitebait fried in batter	600	Shrimp cocktail	346
Rump steak with black pepper sauce	660	Chicken casserole	160
French fries	210	New potatoes	60
Peas	20	French beans	4
Queen pudding	480	Fresh fruit salad	88
Custard	90		
Stilton & biscuits & butter	570	Camembert & biscuits	270
Coffee & cream 1 sugar	60	Black coffee	2
Total	2690	*Total*	930

These menus are included to show how being aware of different calorie values can help you reduce your intake without great changes to the amount of food or the types of meals you eat.

The first example is for a business lunch or evening dinner - here the second menu contains nearly 60% less calories than the first.

The second examples are chosen to show different intakes of food during the day in an office or workplace.

Again there is not a great deal of difference in the amount or type of food but the second menu contains less than half the calories of the first.   When you plan your diet try to keep your pattern of eating the same and choose equivalent foods with lower calorie values.

Menu 1	calories per serving	*Menu 2*	calories per serving
Elevenses		*Elevenses*	
Tea with milk & sugar	50	Black coffee or lemon tea	4
2 chocolate biscuits	200	1 plain digestive biscuit	100
Lunch		*Lunch*	
White roll with chicken and		Wholemeal roll with cottage	
mayonnaise filling	390	cheese & chives filling -	
Cream of tomato soup	308	no butter	147
Chocolate eclair	155	Cup of minestrone soup	156
Coca cola	88	Banana	50
		Diet coke/pepsi etc	1
Tea		*Tea*	
Tea with milk & sugar	50	Black coffee or lemon tea	4
2 chocolate biscuits	200	1 plain digestive biscuit	100
Total	1441	**Total**	562

Guidelines for

1 Assess your average calorie intake over the past weeks or month. Is your weight generally increasing, decreasing or staying the same?

2 To start a reducing diet subtract 250-500 calories from your previous daily average; use this for the first week. Then reduce your calorie intake further. Never reduce your average to less than 1000 calories per day. Remember to allow calories for sauces and dressing and methods of food preparation eg frying.

3 Monitor your weight loss with a chart and twice weekly weights. If possible weigh yourself in the morning after opening your bowels with no clothes on. Slow weight loss of 2-3 lbs every 3-4 weeks is more successful for maintaining weight loss. Crash dieting does not work for long term weight loss.

4 Some people find a weekly goal for their calorie intake easier to adapt to than a daily goal, eating more at weekends and less on weekdays or vice versa. You must be reasonable and not eat all your calorie allowance in two days and starve for five.

5 Be sure to maintain variety in your diet and try to adhere to recommended proportions of proteins, carbohydrates and fats.

6 Cut down on alcohol, sweets, biscuits and cake and added sugar, also reduce your intake of red meat and

calorie controlled diets

dairy products eating more vegetables and cereals. Aim to make these changes in your diet permanent ones.

7 Increase your fibre intake to help stave off feelings of hunger and keep your bowels regular. Remember that increasing fibre intake means you need to increase fluid intake too.

8 It is advisable when planning a calorie controlled diet for more than a week or so to supplement your diet with a good daily multivitamin and mineral tablet.

9 If you wish to exercise with a calorie controlled diet do not start the new exercise programme and diet at the same time. Delay one for a week. If you want to attend a gym or fitness class remember you may need to increase your calorie intake to provide extra energy. Do not further decrease calories at this point.

10 Remember that even if you are ill with a simple cold or flu you may need to increase your calorie intake. Some people find that restricting calories too drastically causes headaches, lethargy and irritability. Watch out for signs that you are not allowing your body adequate calories for the work it has to do.

11 Above all make sure you are planning a diet you have some chance of enjoying. A diet which makes you miserable will not succeed.

Section 1

Food listings A-Z

FOODS	Calories per		Carbohydrates per		Fat per		Fibre per		Protein per	
	oz	100g	oz	100g	oz	100g	oz	100g	oz	100g
Advocaat	78	270	8	28	2	6	0	0	1	5
Ale, brown	8	28	1	3	0	0	0	0	0	0
Ale, pale	9	32	1	2	0	0	0	0	0	0
Ale, strong	21	70	2	6	0	0	0	0	0	1
Alfalfa	23	79	2	7	1	2	0	0	3	9
All bran cereal	77	273	12	43	2	6	8	27	4	15
Almond paste [marzipan]	127	443	14	49	7	25	2	6	2	9
Almonds, ground	181	633	1	4	16	58	2	6	7	25
Almonds, kernel	161	565	1	4	15	54	4	15	5	17
Apple, baked in skin	9	32	2	8	0	0	1	2	0	0
Apple chutney	55	190	14	51	0	0	1	2	0	1
Apple crumble, frozen	72	252	12	43	2	9	0	0	1	3
Apple, dessert	14	48	3	12	0	0	1	2	0	1
Apple, fresh peeled & cored	13	46	3	12	0	0	1	2	0	0
Apple juice	13	45	3	12	0	0	0	0	0	0
Apple pie filling, tinned	18	62	5	16	0	0	0	0	0	0
Apple pie, pastry top only	51	180	8	28	2	8	1	3	1	3
Apple sauce	27	94	7	24	0	0	0	0	0	0
Apple, stewed no sugar	9	32	2	8	0	0	1	2	0	0
Apple strudel, frozen	79	276	10	36	0	0	4	14	1	3

FOODS	Calories per oz	Calories per 100g	Carbohydrates per oz	Carbohydrates per 100g	Fat per oz	Fat per 100g	Fibre per oz	Fibre per 100g	Protein per oz	Protein per 100g
Apple & blackberry pie filling, tinned	19	67	5	17	0	0	0	0	0	1
Apple & raspberry pie filling, tinned	18	62	5	16	0	0	0	0	0	1
Apricot, fresh	8	28	2	7	0	0	1	3	0	1
Apricot, cooked no sugar	7	23	2	6	0	0	1	2	0	0
Apricot, tinned in juice	13	44	3	11	0	0	0	0	0	1
Apricot, tinned in syrup	20	71	5	18	0	0	0	0	0	1
Apricot, dried	52	182	12	43	0	0	7	24	1	5
Apricot jam	72	253	19	67	0	0	0	0	0	0
Ardennes paté	99	348	1	4	9	32	0	0	3	12
Artichoke, globe boiled	4	15	1	3	0	0	0	0	0	1
Artichoke, Jerusalem boiled	5	18	1	3	0	0	0	0	0	2
Asparagus, fresh boiled	5	18	0	1	0	0	1	2	1	3
Aubergine, raw	4	15	1	3	0	0	1	3	0	1
Avocado pear	64	223	1	2	6	22	1	2	1	4
Bacon, gammon lean grilled	49	172	0	0	1	5	0	0	9	31
Bacon rashers, lean fried	95	332	0	0	6	22	0	0	9	33
Bacon rashers, lean grilled	83	292	0	0	5	19	0	0	9	31
Baguettes, frozen bread	73	255	16	57	0	1	1	3	2	7
Baking powder	47	160	11	38	0	0	0	0	1	5

FOODS	Calories per oz	100g	Carbohydrates per oz	100g	Fat per oz	100g	Fibre per oz	100g	Protein per oz	100g
Banana, fresh peeled	22	80	5	19	0	0	1	3	0	1
Banana mousse, frozen	47	163	7	23	2	7	0	0	1	4
Barley, pearl boiled	30	105	6	22	0	1	1	2	1	4
Bean salad	20	70	4	13	0	1	1	5	1	4
Beans baked in tomato sauce	18	64	3	10	0	1	2	7	1	5
Beans baked & pork sausage	39	136	5	16	2	6	1	2	2	6
Beans, broad fresh boiled	14	48	2	7	0	1	1	3	1	4
Beans, broad frozen	14	48	2	7	0	1	1	4	1	4
Beans, broad tinned	14	50	2	6	0	1	1	5	2	6
Beans, butter boiled	27	95	5	17	0	0	1	5	2	7
Beans, butter tinned	17	59	3	9	0	0	1	5	2	6
Beans, curried	29	101	6	21	0	0	2	7	1	5
Beans, french fresh boiled	2	7	0	1	0	0	1	3	0	1
Beans, red kidney tinned	29	101	5	17	0	1	3	9	2	8
Beans, runner boiled	5	19	1	3	0	0	1	3	1	2
Beansprouts, fresh	11	40	2	6	0	0	0	0	1	4
Beansprouts, tinned	3	9	0	1	0	0	1	3	1	2
Beaujolais wine	19	68	0	0	0	0	0	0	0	0
Beef, corned	61	217	0	0	3	12	0	0	8	25
Beef dripping	252	891	0	0	28	99	0	0	0	0

FOODS	Calories per oz	Calories per 100g	Carbohydrates per oz	Carbohydrates per 100g	Fat per oz	Fat per 100g	Fibre per oz	Fibre per 100g	Protein per oz	Protein per 100g
Beef, mince stewed	65	229	0	0	4	15	0	0	7	23
Beef & onion pasty	80	281	9	30	4	15	1	1	2	7
Beef, roast sirloin, lean & fat	81	284	0	0	6	21	0	0	7	24
Beef, roast topside, lean & fat	61	214	0	0	3	12	0	0	8	27
Beef, silverside boiled lean	49	173	0	0	1	5	0	0	9	32
Beef spread	43	149	1	4	2	8	0	0	5	16
Beef steak rump grilled lean	48	168	0	0	2	6	0	0	8	29
Beef steak stewed lean & fat	64	220	0	0	3	11	0	0	9	30
Beef stew	34	119	1	4	2	8	0	0	3	10
Beef stew & dumplings	42	147	4	13	2	7	0	0	2	8
Beef stock cubes	78	273	2	7	6	20	0	0	5	17
Beef suet, shredded	230	813	3	12	25	85	0	0	0	0
Beefburgers, low fat	57	198	1	3	4	13	0	0	5	18
Beefburgers with onion	85	296	2	7	7	24	0	0	4	15
Beefsteak pie, frozen	77	268	6	22	5	17	0	0	3	9
Beefsteak & kidney pie	71	250	6	20	4	15	0	0	3	9
Beefsteak & kidney pie, frozen	92	254	6	23	4	15	0	0	3	10
Beer, best bitter	9	33	1	3	0	0	0	0	0	0
Beer, brown ale	8	28	1	3	0	0	0	0	0	0
Beer, pale ale	9	32	1	2	0	0	0	0	0	0

FOODS	Calories per oz	100g	Carbohydrates per oz	100g	Fat per oz	100g	Fibre per oz	100g	Protein per oz	100g
Beer, stout, bottled	10	37	1	4	0	0	0	0	0	0
Beer, strong ale	21	70	2	6	0	0	0	0	0	1
Beer, Yorkshire bitter	12	42	1	3	0	0	0	0	0	0
Beetroot, boiled fresh	13	44	3	10	0	0	1	3	1	3
Beetroot in vinegar, pickle	16	57	4	13	0	0	1	3	1	2
Bilberries	16	56	4	14	0	0	0	0	0	1
Bitter lemon drink	10	34	3	9	0	0	0	0	0	0
Black Forest gateau	90	319	10	35	5	19	0	1	1	4
Black pudding, fried	87	305	4	15	6	22	0	0	4	13
Blackberries, fresh raw	8	29	2	5	0	0	2	7	0	1
Blackberries, stewed no sugar	7	25	2	6	0	0	2	6	0	1
Blackberry & apple pie filling, tinned	19	67	5	17	0	0	0	0	0	1
Blackcurrants, fresh	8	28	2	7	0	0	2	9	0	1
Blackcurrant squash	82	290	22	76	0	0	0	0	0	0
Blackcurrants, tinned in syrup	17	60	4	15	0	0	1	3	0	1
Blackeye beans	38	132	7	23	0	0	2	7	3	10
Bloater, grilled filleted	72	251	0	0	5	17	0	0	7	23
Bolognaise sauce	17	59	2	8	1	3	0	0	1	3
Bournvita powder gross	108	377	23	79	1	5	0	0	2	9
Bovril meat extract gross	50	174	1	3	0	1	0	0	11	40

FOODS	Calories per oz	100g	Carbohydrates per oz	100g	Fat per oz	100g	Fibre per oz	100g	Protein per oz	100g
Brain, calf boiled	40	150	0	0	3	10	0	0	3	12
Brain, lamb boiled	35	125	0	0	3	10	0	0	3	12
Bramble jelly	72	253	19	66	0	0	0	1	0	0
Bran flakes	94	329	20	72	1	2	4	15	3	9
Bran, wheat	59	206	8	27	2	6	13	44	4	14
Brandy 70% proof neat	63	222	0	0	0	0	0	0	0	0
Brawn, cooked meat	45	150	0	0	3	10	0	0	4	12
Brazil nuts	177	619	1	4	18	62	3	9	3	12
Bread, brown	71	249	13	52	1	2	1	5	2	8
Bread, garlic white	117	409	14	47	6	22	1	2	2	8
Bread, Hovis	69	243	13	46	1	3	1	5	3	10
Bread, white [1 thin slice = 1 oz]	67	233	14	50	1	2	1	3	2	8
Bread, wholemeal	69	242	14	48	1	2	2	9	3	10
Bread, white fried	159	558	15	51	11	37	1	2	2	8
Bread, white toasted	85	297	19	65	1	2	1	3	3	10
Bread rolls, crusty, brown	85	290	15	55	1	3	2	6	3	12
Bread rolls, crusty, white	85	290	15	55	1	3	1	3	3	12
Bread rolls soft, brown	81	282	14	48	2	6	2	5	3	12
Bread rolls soft, white	87	305	15	54	2	7	1	3	3	10
Bread currant	71	250	15	52	1	3	1	2	2	6

FOODS	Calories per oz	100g	Carbohydrates per oz	100g	Fat per oz	100g	Fibre per oz	100g	Protein per oz	100g
Bread, malt	81	287	17	61	1	3	0	0	2	8
Bread, soda	75	264	16	56	1	2	1	2	2	8
Bread sauce	36	127	5	18	1	4	0	0	1	5
Bread and butter pudding	45	159	5	15	2	8	0	1	2	5
Breadcrumbs, white dried	100	354	22	78	1	2	1	3	3	12
Breton paté	90	318	2	6	8	28	0	0	4	13
Brie	89	310	0	0	7	24	0	0	6	20
Broad beans, frozen	14	48	2	7	0	1	1	4	1	4
Broad beans, tinned	14	50	2	6	0	1	1	5	2	6
Broccoli spears boiled	5	18	0	2	0	0	1	4	1	3
Broccoli spears frozen	9	32	1	5	0	0	0	0	1	3
Broccoli mornay	26	91	2	6	2	6	0	1	1	4
Brown sauce, bottled	32	112	8	27	0	1	0	0	0	1
Brussels sprouts, fresh boiled	5	18	0	2	0	0	0	0	1	3
Brussels sprouts, frozen	6	20	1	2	0	0	1	3	1	3
Brussels paté	98	345	0	1	9	33	0	0	4	13
Bubble & Squeak	43	149	6	22	2	6	0	0	1	3
Buns, currant	85	298	15	52	2	8	1	2	2	8
Burgundy wine	19	68	0	0	0	0	0	0	0	0
Butter	210	740	0	0	25	85	0	0	0	0

FOODS	Calories per		Carbohydrates per		Fat per		Fibre per		Protein per	
	oz	100g	oz	100g	oz	100g	oz	100g	oz	100g
Butter beans, dried	77	273	14	50	0	1	5	20	5	20
Butter peanut	169	596	4	13	14	51	2	8	7	24
Cabbage, frozen	6	21	1	4	0	0	1	3	0	1
Cabbage, green or savoy boiled	3	9	0	1	0	0	1	3	0	1
Cabbage, spring boiled	2	7	0	1	0	0	1	2	0	2
Cabbage, winter boiled	4	15	1	2	0	0	1	3	0	2
Caerphilly cheese	105	367	0	0	9	30	0	0	7	23
Calf brain, boiled	43	152	0	0	3	11	0	0	4	13
Camembert	82	289	0	0	7	24	0	0	5	19
Caramel dessert	28	97	5	19	0	1	0	0	1	4
Caramel sauce	87	306	23	80	0	0	0	0	0	0
Carp, fresh	26	92	0	0	1	2	0	0	5	18
Carrots, fresh boiled	6	20	1	5	0	0	1	3	0	1
Carrots, frozen	7	24	2	6	0	0	1	3	0	1
Carrots, tinned	5	19	1	4	0	0	1	4	0	1
Cashew nuts	161	564	6	21	13	46	2	7	5	19
Cauliflower, frozen	4	13	0	2	0	0	1	2	1	2

FOODS	Calories per oz	Calories per 100g	Carbohydrates per oz	Carbohydrates per 100g	Fat per oz	Fat per 100g	Fibre per oz	Fibre per 100g	Protein per oz	Protein per 100g
Cauliflower, boiled	3	9	0	1	0	0	1	2	0	2
Cauliflower florets, frozen	3	10	0	1	0	0	1	2	0	2
Cauliflower cheese	29	100	2	8	2	6	0	1	2	6
Cauliflower quiche	70	246	5	19	5	16	1	2	2	7
Celeriac, boiled	4	14	1	2	0	0	1	5	0	2
Celery, fresh raw	3	10	1	2	0	0	1	2	0	1
Celery, boiled	1	5	0	1	0	0	1	2	0	0
Champagne	22	76	0	1	0	0	0	0	0	0
Chapatis, no fat	60	200	10	45	0	1	1	3	2	5
Chapatis, with fat	95	335	15	50	5	15	1	4	2	8
Cheddar cheese	115	406	0	0	10	34	0	0	7	26
Cheese and onion crisps	143	500	11	39	10	37	3	12	2	6
Cheese biscuits	143	505	15	53	8	30	0	0	3	10
Cheesecake	100	420	7	25	10	35	0	0	1	5
Cheese, macaroni	50	174	4	15	3	10	0	0	2	7
Cheese, macaroni tinned	34	118	4	13	2	6	0	0	1	5
Cheese pudding	48	170	2	8	3	11	0	0	3	10
Cheese sauce	36	127	4	13	2	6	0	0	2	6
Cheese soufflé	70	250	3	9	5	20	0	0	3	12
Cheese spread	81	283	0	1	7	23	0	0	5	18

FOODS	Calories per oz	100g	Carbohydrates per oz	100g	Fat per oz	100g	Fibre per oz	100g	Protein per oz	100g
Cheese and mushroom pizza	76	267	11	40	2	7	0	0	4	13
Cheese and onion pizza	67	233	7	23	4	13	0	1	2	8
Cheese and tomato pizza	75	262	10	36	2	8	0	0	4	13
Cheeseburger frozen	76	266	3	10	5	19	0	0	4	16
Cherries eating, raw	13	47	3	12	0	0	1	2	0	1
Cherries, stewed, no sugar	11	39	3	10	0	0	0	1	0	1
Cherries, glacé	60	212	15	55	0	0	1	2	0	1
Cherry brandy	73	255	10	35	0	0	0	0	0	0
Cherry pie filling, tinned	27	94	7	24	0	0	0	0	0	1
Cherryade, carbonated	7	23	2	6	0	0	0	0	0	0
Cheshire cheese	106	371	0	0	9	31	0	0	7	24
Chestnuts, shelled	49	170	10	37	1	3	2	7	1	2
Chick peas	44	154	7	24	1	3	1	4	3	10
Chick peas, cooked dahl	40	145	6	22	1	3	2	6	2	8
Chicken, boiled meat	52	183	0	0	2	7	0	0	8	29
Chicken curry, tinned	28	98	2	6	1	4	0	0	3	9
Chicken liver, fried	55	194	1	3	3	10	0	0	6	20
Chicken liver paté	53	186	2	8	3	10	0	0	5	17
Chicken noodle soup, as served	6	20	1	4	0	0	0	0	0	1
Chicken quiche	68	239	6	19	4	15	0	1	3	9

FOODS	Calories per		Carbohydrates per		Fat per		Fibre per		Protein per	
	oz	100g	oz	100g	oz	100g	oz	100g	oz	100g
Chicken, roast, no skin	42	148	0	0	2	5	0	0	7	25
Chicken, roast with skin	61	216	0	0	4	15	0	0	7	25
Chicken spread	52	181	1	2	3	11	0	0	5	18
Chicken spring roll	51	180	6	22	2	8	0	0	2	6
Chicken stock cubes	81	285	1	5	6	21	0	0	5	19
Chicken supreme, tinned	45	156	1	4	3	10	0	0	4	13
Chicken and ham paste	64	225	1	2	5	16	0	0	5	19
Chicory, cooked	5	17	1	3	0	0	0	0	0	1
Chicory, raw	3	9	0	2	0	0	0	0	0	1
Chilli beans	32	112	6	22	0	1	1	5	2	6
Chilli con carne	33	114	1	3	2	7	3	9	3	11
Chips, potato	70	250	10	35	3	10	0	0	1	5
Choc Ice, vanilla	75	263	6	21	5	19	1	1	1	4
Chocolate, milk	149	529	17	60	8	30	0	0	2	10
Chocolate, plain	148	525	18	65	8	24	0	0	1	5
Chocolate biscuits, all over	150	524	20	65	8	28	1	3	2	6
Chocolate digestive biscuits	141	493	20	65	8	25	1	3	2	7
Chocolate drinking, made-up	28	99	3	12	1	4	0	0	1	4
Chocolate drinking powder	106	374	23	80	2	6	0	0	1	5
Chocolate ice cream	83	290	7	26	6	20	0	0	1	4

FOODS	Calories per oz	Calories per 100g	Carbohydrates per oz	Carbohydrates per 100g	Fat per oz	Fat per 100g	Fibre per oz	Fibre per 100g	Protein per oz	Protein per 100g
Chocolate mousse, frozen	46	161	6	23	2	7	0	0	2	7
Chocolate sauce	90	318	23	80	0	1	0	0	1	2
Chocolate sponge	100	351	17	58	4	13	0	0	1	5
Chocolate supreme dessert	33	115	5	17	1	5	0	0	1	3
Choux pastry, cooked	94	330	9	30	6	20	0	1	2	10
Christmas pudding	87	304	14	50	3	12	1	2	1	5
Chutney, apple	55	193	14	51	0	0	1	2	0	1
Chutney, tomato	44	154	11	40	0	0	1	2	0	1
Cider, dry	10	36	1	3	0	0	0	0	0	0
Cider, strong	10	35	1	2	0	0	0	0	0	0
Cider, medium sweet	12	43	2	6	0	0	0	0	0	0
Cider, sweet	12	42	1	4	0	0	0	0	0	0
Cider, vintage	29	101	2	7	0	0	0	0	0	0
Cinnamon	95	337	23	80	1	2	6	20	1	5
Claret wine	19	68	0	0	0	0	0	0	0	0
Coalfish [Saithe] steamed	28	99	0	0	0	0	0	0	7	25
Cob [hazel] nuts	106	375	2	7	10	35	2	6	2	8
Coca-cola	11	39	3	11	0	0	0	0	0	0
Cockles, boiled	14	48	0	0	0	0	0	0	3	11
Cocktail cherries	48	168	13	44	0	0	0	0	0	0

FOODS	Calories per oz	Calories per 100g	Carbohydrates per oz	Carbohydrates per 100g	Fat per oz	Fat per 100g	Fibre per oz	Fibre per 100g	Protein per oz	Protein per 100g
Cocktail gherkins	3	9	1	2	0	0	0	0	0	1
Cocktail olives	31	111	1	5	3	10	0	0	0	1
Cocktail onions	3	10	1	2	0	0	0	0	0	1
Cocktail sausage	91	319	4	13	7	25	0	0	4	12
Cocoa	91	317	3	12	6	22	0	0	6	20
Coconut cake	119	416	14	50	7	24	0	0	2	6
Coconut, dessicated	173	604	2	6	18	62	7	24	2	6
Coconut, fresh	100	351	1	4	10	36	4	14	1	3
Coconut, milk	6	21	1	5	0	0	0	0	0	0
Coconut slice	100	351	20	71	2	8	0	0	1	3
Cod, baked or grilled	27	95	0	0	0	1	0	0	6	20
Cod fillets, fresh	22	78	0	0	0	1	0	0	5	18
Cod in batter, fresh	70	244	4	13	5	16	0	0	4	13
Cod in breadcrumbs	61	212	4	14	4	13	0	0	3	11
Cod in butter sauce	25	90	1	3	1	4	0	0	3	10
Cod fishcakes	62	216	5	19	3	11	0	0	3	11
Cod fishfingers	52	185	5	20	2	10	0	0	3	10
Cod in parsley sauce	23	80	1	2	1	4	0	0	3	10
Cod, poached	27	94	0	0	0	1	0	0	6	21
Cod, smoked poached	29	100	0	0	0	2	0	0	6	20

FOODS	Calories per oz	Calories per 100g	Carbohydrates per oz	Carbohydrates per 100g	Fat per oz	Fat per 100g	Fibre per oz	Fibre per 100g	Protein per oz	Protein per 100g
Cod, steamed	24	83	0	0	0	1	0	0	5	20
Cod steaks in light batter	69	241	3	11	5	17	0	0	3	12
Cod liver oil	257	899	0	0	29	100	0	0	0	0
Cod roe hard, fried	57	202	1	3	3	12	0	0	6	21
Coffee and chicory essence	62	218	16	56	0	0	0	0	0	2
Coffee, ground roasted	80	280	8	30	4	15	0	0	3	10
Coffee, black	0	0	0	0	0	0	0	0	0	0
Coffee, instant powder	30	100	3	10	0	0	0	0	4	15
Coffee whitener, powder gross	155	540	15	55	10	35	0	0	1	3
Cola see also Coca-cola	12	42	3	11	0	0	0	0	0	0
Cola diet	0	0	0	0	0	0	0	0	0	0
Coleslaw salad	34	120	2	7	3	10	1	2	0	1
Coley, fresh or frozen	28	99	0	0	0	1	0	0	7	23
Corn cobs, baby, frozen	8	28	1	3	0	0	1	5	1	3
Corn on the cob, boiled	35	123	7	23	1	2	1	5	1	4
Corn flakes	105	370	25	85	0	2	3	10	2	10
Corn oil	255	900	0	0	28	100	0	0	0	0
Corn relish	34	118	9	30	0	0	1	2	0	1
Corned beef	61	217	0	0	3	12	0	0	8	25
Cornflour	95	334	25	87	0	0	0	0	0	0

FOODS	Calories per oz	100g	Carbohydrates per oz	100g	Fat per oz	100g	Fibre per oz	100g	Protein per oz	100g
Cornish pasty	95	330	9	30	6	20	0	0	2	8
Coronation chicken salad	51	179	4	15	3	11	0	0	2	6
Cottage cheese	28	98	1	3	1	4	0	0	4	13
Cottage pie	42	148	4	14	2	8	0	0	2	6
Courgettes, raw	7	25	1	5	0	0	0	0	0	2
Courgettes, sliced cooked	5	16	1	4	0	0	0	0	0	1
Crab bisque soup	12	41	1	4	0	1	0	0	1	3
Crab, boiled shelled	35	125	0	0	1	5	0	0	6	20
Crab paste	53	186	1	3	3	12	0	0	5	18
Crab spread	38	134	1	5	2	6	0	0	4	14
Crab tinned	25	80	0	0	0	1	0	0	5	18
Cranberries, fresh	4	15	1	4	0	0	1	4	0	0
Cranberry sauce	39	137	10	36	0	0	0	0	0	0
Cream, clotted	156	550	0	1	17	60	0	0	0	1
Cream, double	128	447	1	2	15	50	0	0	0	2
Cream, single	55	193	1	4	5	19	0	0	1	3
Cream, soured	54	190	1	3	5	18	0	0	1	3
Cream, tinned sterilised	68	240	1	4	7	25	0	0	1	3
Cream, whipping	103	364	1	3	11	39	0	0	1	2
Cream of asparagus soup, tinned	16	55	1	4	1	4	0	0	0	1

FOODS	Calories per oz	Calories per 100g	Carbohydrates per oz	Carbohydrates per 100g	Fat per oz	Fat per 100g	Fibre per oz	Fibre per 100g	Protein per oz	Protein per 100g
Cream of celery soup, tinned	15	52	1	4	1	4	0	0	0	1
Cream of chicken soup, tinned	17	61	1	5	1	4	0	0	1	2
Cream of mushroom soup, tinned	15	54	1	5	1	4	0	0	0	1
Cream of tomato soup, tinned	22	77	3	11	1	4	0	0	0	1
Cream cheese	125	440	0	0	15	50	0	0	1	3
Cream crackers	125	440	20	68	5	16	1	3	3	10
Creamed rice	25	88	5	16	0	2	0	0	1	3
Creme Caramel, chilled	31	110	6	21	0	2	0	0	1	4
Cress, mustard	3	10	0	1	0	0	1	4	0	2
Cress, water raw	4	14	0	1	0	0	1	3	1	3
Crisps potato	143	500	11	39	10	37	3	12	2	6
Crispbread, rye	92	321	20	71	1	2	3	12	3	9
Crispbread, wheat	110	390	10	40	2	8	1	5	15	45
Croissants	121	424	13	46	7	24	0	0	3	9
Crumpets	49	170	11	37	0	0	1	2	2	7
Cucumber, fresh	3	10	1	2	0	0	0	0	0	1
Cucumber, pickled	8	29	2	7	0	0	0	0	0	1
Curacoa	89	311	8	28	0	0	0	0	0	0
Currant bun	85	298	15	52	2	8	1	2	2	8
Currants, black raw	8	28	2	7	0	0	2	10	0	1

FOODS	Calories per oz	Calories per 100g	Carbohydrates per oz	Carbohydrates per 100g	Fat per oz	Fat per 100g	Fibre per oz	Fibre per 100g	Protein per oz	Protein per 100g
Currants, black stewed	7	24	2	6	0	0	2	7	0	1
Currants, dried	70	245	20	65	0	0	2	7	0	2
Currants, red raw	6	21	1	4	0	0	2	8	0	1
Currants, red stewed	5	18	1	4	0	0	2	7	0	1
Currants, white raw	7	26	2	6	0	0	2	7	0	1
Currants, white stewed	6	22	1	5	0	0	2	6	0	1
Curried beans	29	101	6	21	0	0	2	7	1	5
Curry powder	66	233	7	26	3	11	0	0	3	10
Curry powder, hot vindaloo	89	313	11	38	4	13	5	17	4	13
Curry powder, medium Madras	89	311	11	39	4	12	5	16	4	13
Curry powder, mild Korma	85	296	10	36	3	12	5	19	4	12
Curry sauce, tinned	15	52	3	10	0	1	0	0	0	1
Custard, egg	34	118	3	11	2	6	0	0	2	6
Custard, instant made-up	21	74	4	15	0	1	0	0	0	1
Custard powder	100	354	26	92	0	1	0	0	0	1
Custard tart	82	287	8	30	5	17	0	1	2	6
Custard topping, made-up	27	95	4	13	1	4	0	0	1	3

FOODS	Calories per oz	Calories per 100g	Carbohydrates per oz	Carbohydrates per 100g	Fat per oz	Fat per 100g	Fibre per oz	Fibre per 100g	Protein per oz	Protein per 100g
Dahl Bengal gram red, raw	90	320	14	50	2	6	4	15	6	20
Dahl channa	30	100	3	10	1	5	1	5	2	5
Dahl cooked	40	145	6	22	1	3	2	6	2	8
Damsons, raw	11	38	3	10	0	0	1	4	0	1
Damsons stewed no sugar	9	32	2	8	0	0	1	4	0	0
Damson jam	73	254	19	66	0	0	0	0	0	0
Danish Blue cheese	97	342	0	0	8	30	0	0	5	20
Dates	60	213	16	55	0	0	2	8	1	2
Dessert delights, made-up	40	142	6	20	2	6	0	0	1	3
Diet cola	0	0	0	0	0	0	0	0	0	0
Digestive biscuits, chocolate	141	493	20	65	8	25	1	3	2	7
Digestive biscuits, plain	135	471	19	66	6	20	2	5	3	10
Dover sole, fresh	23	81	0	0	0	1	0	0	5	18
Dripping, beef	252	891	0	0	28	99	0	0	0	0
Dry ginger ale	7	24	2	7	0	0	0	0	0	0
Duck, roast meat only	55	190	0	0	3	10	0	0	7	25
Duck, roast meat fat, skin	95	340	0	0	8	30	0	0	6	20
Duck and orange paté	78	274	1	3	7	24	0	0	4	13
Dumplings	60	210	7	25	3	12	0	1	1	3

FOODS	Calories per		Carbohydrates per		Fat per		Fibre per		Protein per	
	oz	100g	oz	100g	oz	100g	oz	100g	oz	100g
Edam cheese	86	305	0	0	7	23	0	0	7	25
Eddoes, cooked	52	181	12	42	0	1	0	0	1	3
Eel, fresh	66	231	0	0	6	19	0	0	4	14
Eel, stewed	55	200	0	0	4	13	0	0	6	20
Egg custard	34	118	3	11	2	6	0	0	2	6
Eggplant, raw	4	14	1	3	0	0	1	3	0	1
Eggs, raw or boiled	42	148	0	0	3	10	0	0	3	12
Eggs, dried gross	161	564	0	0	12	45	0	0	12	45
Eggs, fried	66	232	0	0	6	20	0	0	4	15
Eggs, omelette	54	190	0	0	5	15	0	0	3	10
Eggs, scotch	80	279	3	12	6	20	0	0	3	10
Eggs, scrambled	70	246	0	0	6	20	0	0	3	10
Eggs, white raw	10	36	0	0	0	0	0	0	3	10
Eggs, yolk raw	95	340	0	0	9	30	0	0	5	16
Emmental cheese	138	486	0	0	8	30	0	0	8	30
Endive, raw	3	11	0	1	0	0	1	2	1	2
Evaporated milk, unsweetened	44	154	3	11	3	9	0	0	2	8

FOODS	Calories per oz	Calories per 100g	Carbohydrates per oz	Carbohydrates per 100g	Fat per oz	Fat per 100g	Fibre per oz	Fibre per 100g	Protein per oz	Protein per 100g
Faggots	75	270	4	15	5	20	0	0	3	11
Fancy iced cake	116	407	19	67	4	15	1	2	1	4
Fennel, cooked	6	22	1	4	0	1	0	0	0	1
Figroll biscuits	97	338	20	69	2	6	2	7	1	4
Figs, fresh	12	41	3	10	0	0	1	3	0	1
Figs dried raw	61	213	15	53	0	0	5	19	1	4
Figs stewed no sugar	34	118	8	30	0	0	3	10	1	2
Fish paste	48	169	1	4	3	10	0	0	4	15
Fish pie	36	128	4	13	2	6	0	0	2	7
Fish stew	35	124	3	10	2	7	0	0	1	5
Fishcakes, frozen	32	112	5	7	0	1	0	0	3	10
Fishcakes, fried	54	188	4	15	3	11	0	0	3	10
Fishfingers, frozen	54	189	5	17	2	8	0	0	4	14
Fishfingers, fried	67	233	5	17	4	13	0	0	4	14
Flaky pastry, cooked	161	565	15	50	12	40	1	2	2	6
Flour, wholemeal stoneground	90	318	19	66	1	2	3	10	4	13
Flour, brown	93	327	20	69	1	2	2	8	4	13
Flour, white plain	100	350	23	80	0	1	1	3	3	10
Flour, self-raising	97	340	22	78	0	1	1	4	3	10
Frankfurters	78	274	1	3	7	25	0	0	3	10

FOODS	Calories per oz	Calories per 100g	Carbohydrates per oz	Carbohydrates per 100g	Fat per oz	Fat per 100g	Fibre per oz	Fibre per 100g	Protein per oz	Protein per 100g
French beans boiled	2	7	0	1	0	0	1	3	0	1
French salad dressing	139	487	0	0	16	55	0	0	0	0
Fried bread	159	558	15	51	11	37	1	2	2	8
Fromage frais, natural	30	106	1	3	2	8	0	0	2	7
Fromage frais, natural very low fat	12	43	1	3	0	0	0	0	2	8
Fruit [see under name]										
Fruit cake, plain	100	354	17	58	4	13	1	3	1	5
Fruit cake, iced	100	352	18	62	4	13	1	3	1	4
Fruit cake, rich	95	337	17	58	4	13	1	3	1	4
Fruit cocktail, chilled	43	149	6	20	2	7	0	0	0	2
Fruit pie, individual	105	370	15	60	4	16	1	3	1	4
Fruit pie, pastry top	51	180	8	28	2	8	1	2	1	2
Fruit salad, tinned in natural juice	14	49	4	13	0	0	0	0	0	0
Fruit sauce, bottled	31	107	8	27	0	0	0	0	0	1
Garden beans, sliced frozen	2	8	0	1	0	0	1	3	0	1
Garibaldi biscuits	111	390	22	77	3	9	0	0	1	4
Garlic [about 5 per oz] raw	33	117	8	27	0	0	0	0	1	4
Garlic mayonnaise	208	734	0	0	23	81	0	0	1	2
Garlic oil dressing	127	443	0	1	14	49	0	0	0	0

FOODS	Calories per		Carbohydrates per		Fat per		Fibre per		Protein per	
	oz	100g	oz	100g	oz	100g	oz	100g	oz	100g
Gazpacho soup, tinned	12	43	3	10	0	0	0	1	0	1
Gelatin	97	338	0	0	0	0	0	0	25	85
Gherkins, pickled	3	9	1	2	0	0	0	0	0	1
Gin 70% proof	63	222	0	0	0	0	0	0	0	0
Ginger ale, dry	7	24	2	7	0	0	0	0	0	0
Ginger beer	14	49	4	13	0	0	0	0	0	0
Ginger, ground	97	342	18	65	2	6	0	0	3	10
Ginger nuts	130	456	25	80	4	15	1	2	2	6
Ginger preserve	72	253	19	67	0	0	0	1	0	0
Ginger root, raw	13	46	2	8	0	1	0	0	0	2
Gingerbread	107	373	18	63	4	13	0	1	2	6
Glacé cherries	60	212	16	56	0	0	1	2	0	1
Globe artichokes, boiled	4	15	1	3	0	0	0	0	0	1
Goats milk	20	71	1	5	1	5	0	0	1	3
Golden syrup	85	298	25	80	0	0	0	0	0	0
Goose, roast	90	319	0	0	6	22	0	0	8	30
Goose, meat only	66	230	0	0	4	15	0	0	8	30
Gooseberries, fresh	5	17	1	3	0	0	1	3	0	1
Gooseberries, stewed no sugar	4	14	1	3	0	0	1	3	0	1
Gooseberry fool	31	110	4	13	2	6	0	0	0	1

FOODS	Calories per		Carbohydrates per		Fat per		Fibre per		Protein per	
	oz	100g	oz	100g	oz	100g	oz	100g	oz	100g
Gooseberry pie	51	180	8	28	2	8	1	2	1	2
Gooseberry pie filling, tinned	20	70	5	18	0	0	0	0	0	0
Gorgonzola cheese	101	355	0	0	8	29	0	0	7	23
Gouda cheese	87	305	0	0	7	23	0	0	7	25
Granadilla [passion fruit]	10	34	2	6	0	0	5	15	1	3
Grapefruit, fresh	6	22	1	5	0	0	0	1	0	1
Grapefruit, tinned in natural juice	10	36	3	9	0	0	0	0	0	0
Grapefruit, tinned in syrup	19	68	5	17	0	0	0	0	0	1
Grapefruit juice, pure	11	40	3	10	0	0	0	0	0	0
Grapenuts	100	355	22	75	1	3	2	7	3	10
Grapes, fresh black	14	51	4	13	0	0	0	0	0	1
Grapes, fresh white	18	63	5	16	0	0	0	1	0	1
Gravy powder	65	228	14	50	0	0	0	0	2	6
Gravy granules, made-up	10	35	1	3	1	3	0	0	0	0
Gravy mix, made-up	4	13	1	3	0	0	0	0	0	0
Green beans, frozen	2	8	0	1	0	0	1	3	0	1
Green split peas, cooked	37	128	6	22	0	1	1	5	3	10
Greengages, fresh	13	47	3	12	0	0	1	3	0	1
Greengages, stewed with sugar	21	75	5	19	0	0	1	2	0	1
Grey mullet	31	109	0	0	1	4	0	0	5	18

COUNT YOUR CALORIES					51

FOODS	Calories per		Carbohydrates per		Fat per		Fibre per		Protein per	
	oz	100g	oz	100g	oz	100g	oz	100g	oz	100g
Grouse, roast	49	173	0	0	2	5	0	0	9	31
Gruyere cheese	126	446	0	0	9	33	0	0	11	38
Guavas	18	62	3	9	0	1	0	0	0	1
Guinness	10	37	1	4	0	0	0	0	0	0
Haddock in batter	70	244	4	13	5	16	0	0	4	13
Haddock in breadcrumbs	55	191	3	11	3	10	0	0	4	15
Haddock fillets, fresh	22	77	0	0	0	1	0	0	5	18
Haddock fillets, frozen	29	102	0	0	0	1	0	0	7	23
Haddock, fried	50	174	1	4	2	8	0	0	6	21
Haddock, steamed	28	98	0	0	0	1	0	0	7	23
Haddock, smoked steamed	29	101	0	0	0	1	0	0	7	23
Haggis, boiled	90	310	5	20	6	22	0	0	3	10
Hake, fresh or frozen	23	79	0	0	0	1	0	0	5	18
Halibut, fresh	34	120	0	0	1	5	0	0	5	18
Halibut, steamed	37	131	0	0	1	4	0	0	7	24
Ham, chopped tinned	33	115	1	3	1	5	0	0	4	15
Ham, smoked	26	91	0	1	0	1	0	0	5	19
Ham and mushroom pizza	67	234	9	32	2	8	0	0	3	11
Ham and pork, chopped	77	270	0	0	7	24	0	0	4	14

FOODS	Calories per oz	100g	Carbohydrates per oz	100g	Fat per oz	100g	Fibre per oz	100g	Protein per oz	100g
Hamburgers, tinned	36	126	2	7	2	8	0	0	2	8
Hare, stewed/jugged	54	192	0	0	2	8	0	0	9	30
Haricot beans, cooked	39	135	6	23	0	1	2	7	3	11
Haricot beans, dried	75	270	13	45	1	2	7	25	6	20
Hazelnuts (cobnuts)	106	375	2	7	10	36	2	6	2	8
Heart, lamb	33	118	0	0	2	6	0	0	5	17
Heart, ox	51	180	0	0	2	6	0	0	9	32
Heart, pig	27	93	0	0	1	3	0	0	5	17
Herring, fresh	66	232	0	0	5	19	0	0	5	17
Herring, fried	67	234	0	2	4	15	0	0	7	23
Herring, grilled	57	199	0	0	4	13	0	0	6	20
Herring roe, soft fried	69	244	1	5	5	16	0	0	6	21
Honey	88	311	23	81	0	0	0	0	0	0
Horlicks, malted milk powder	112	396	21	73	2	10	0	1	4	15
Horseradish sauce	53	185	5	18	3	11	1	2	1	3
Hotpot	35	115	3	10	1	4	0	0	3	10
Hundreds and thousands	107	375	28	99	0	0	0	0	0	0
Huss	35	122	0	0	1	5	0	0	6	20

FOODS	Calories per		Carbohydrates per		Fat per		Fibre per		Protein per	
	oz	100g	oz	100g	oz	100g	oz	100g	oz	100g
Ice cream, dairy	50	170	7	25	2	7	0	0	1	4
Ice cream, non-dairy	48	165	6	20	2	8	0	0	1	3
Ice cream roll, frozen	51	178	9	31	1	5	0	0	1	4
Ice cream, chocolate	83	290	7	26	6	20	0	0	1	4
Iced fruit cake	100	352	18	62	3	12	1	3	1	4
Instant dried milk	101	355	15	53	0	1	0	0	10	36
Irish stew, tinned	27	95	2	6	1	5	0	0	2	8
Irish stew	35	124	3	10	2	7	0	0	1	5
Italian oil dressing	126	444	0	1	14	49	0	0	0	0
Jaffa orange juice	12	43	3	11	0	0	0	0	0	1
Jam, average	75	261	20	69	0	0	0	1	0	0
Jam sponge pudding	97	341	17	59	3	11	0	0	1	4
Jam suet pudding	90	316	17	57	3	10	0	0	1	3
Jam tarts	110	384	18	63	4	15	2	2	1	4
Jellied veal	36	125	0	0	1	3	0	0	7	25
Jelly cubes	77	268	19	66	0	0	0	0	2	6
Jelly, made with water	17	58	4	14	0	0	0	0	0	0
Jelly, made with milk	25	85	5	15	0	2	0	0	1	3
Jelly, mint	78	276	20	72	0	0	0	0	0	0

FOODS	Calories per		Carbohydrates per		Fat per		Fibre per		Protein per	
	oz	100g	oz	100g	oz	100g	oz	100g	oz	100g
Jelly, redcurrant	73	256	19	67	0	0	0	0	0	0
Jerusalem artichokes, boiled	5	18	1	3	0	0	0	0	0	2
Kale, boiled	9	33	2	6	0	0	0	1	1	2
Kedgeree	43	151	3	9	2	7	0	0	4	13
Ketchup, tomato average	35	123	9	29	0	1	0	9	0	1
Kidney beans, red tinned	29	101	5	17	0	1	3	9	2	8
Kidney, ox stewed	49	172	0	0	2	8	0	0	7	26
Kidney, lamb's	45	155	0	0	2	6	0	0	7	25
Kidney, pig stewed	43	153	0	0	2	6	0	0	7	24
Kipper, fresh	61	212	0	0	5	16	0	0	5	17
Kipper, baked	59	205	0	0	3	12	0	0	7	26
Kipper fillets, frozen	59	205	0	0	3	12	0	0	7	26
Kipper fillets, fresh boned	61	212	0	0	5	16	0	0	5	17
Kippered mackerel fillets	70	244	0	0	5	18	0	0	6	21
Kiwi fruit	18	63	5	16	0	0	0	0	0	1
Kumquats	23	80	5	19	0	0	0	0	1	2
Kohlrabi, raw	7	24	1	5	0	0	0	0	0	1

FOODS	Calories per oz	Calories per 100g	Carbohydrates per oz	Carbohydrates per 100g	Fat per oz	Fat per 100g	Fibre per oz	Fibre per 100g	Protein per oz	Protein per 100g
Ladies fingers [Okra]	5	17	1	2	0	0	1	3	1	2
Lager bottled/canned	8	29	0	2	0	0	0	0	0	0
Lager, Dutch	8	27	1	2	0	0	0	0	0	0
Lager, German	11	40	1	3	0	0	0	0	0	0
Lamb chops, grilled lean & fat	100	355	0	0	8	30	0	0	7	25
Lamb cutlets	105	370	0	0	9	31	0	0	7	23
Lamb, roast breast	116	410	0	0	11	37	0	0	5	19
Lamb, roast leg	76	266	0	0	5	18	0	0	7	26
Lamb, roast shoulder	90	316	0	0	8	26	0	0	6	20
Lamb, scrag stewed	83	292	0	0	6	21	0	0	7	26
Lamb's heart	33	118	0	0	2	6	0	0	5	17
Lamb's kidney	44	155	0	0	2	6	0	0	7	25
Lamb's tongue, stewed	82	289	0	0	7	24	0	0	5	18
Lard	252	891	0	0	28	99	0	0	0	0
Lasagne, egg raw	95	337	21	73	1	2	1	4	3	12
Lasagne, seafood chilled	34	118	3	11	2	6	0	0	2	6
Lasagne, vegetable frozen	24	85	3	9	1	3	1	1	2	6
Laver bread	15	52	0	2	1	4	3	3	1	3
Leaf spinach, frozen	9	31	1	5	0	0	6	6	1	3
Leek, boiled	7	24	1	5	0	0	4	4	1	2

FOODS	Calories per oz	100g	Carbohydrates per oz	100g	Fat per oz	100g	Fibre per oz	100g	Protein per oz	100g
Lemon, fresh	4	15	1	3	0	0	1	5	0	1
Lemon curd	83	290	19	67	1	4	0	0	0	1
Lemon juice	2	7	0	2	0	0	0	0	0	0
Lemon or Dover sole fillets, fresh	23	81	0	0	0	1	0	0	5	18
Lemon or Dover sole, fried	61	216	3	9	4	13	0	0	5	16
Lemon or Dover sole, steamed	25	90	0	0	0	1	0	0	6	20
Lemon meringue pie	92	323	13	46	4	15	0	1	1	5
Lemon squash, high juice undiluted	42	148	11	39	0	0	0	0	0	0
Lemon whole drink, undiluted	29	103	8	27	0	0	0	0	0	0
Lemonade, carbonated	6	22	2	6	0	0	0	0	0	0
Lemonade, chilled	13	46	3	12	0	0	0	0	0	0
Lemonade shandy	3	16	1	4	0	0	0	0	0	0
Lentils, boiled	31	111	5	17	0	0	1	4	3	10
Lentil soup	11	38	2	7	0	0	0	0	1	2
Lentils, split	86	304	15	53	0	1	3	12	7	24
Lettuce, round/cos/crisp fresh	3	12	0	1	0	0	0	2	0	1
Limes	10	36	2	6	1	2	0	0	0	1
Lime juice cordial, neat	27	97	7	25	0	0	0	0	0	0
Lime marmalade	72	252	19	67	0	0	0	1	0	0
Lincoln biscuits	138	482	20	70	6	21	0	0	2	7

FOODS	Calories per		Carbohydrates per		Fat per		Fibre per		Protein per	
	oz	100g	oz	100g	oz	100g	oz	100g	oz	100g
Liver, calf fried	73	256	2	7	5	15	0	0	8	27
Liver, chicken fried	55	194	1	3	3	12	0	0	6	21
Liver, duck	50	176	0	1	2	8	0	0	7	25
Liver, lamb fried	66	232	1	4	4	14	0	0	7	23
Liver, pig	53	188	1	4	2	8	0	0	7	26
Liver sausage	65	230	2	8	5	17	0	0	4	13
Liver, turkey	48	169	0	1	2	6	0	0	8	27
Lobster bisque soup, tinned	18	62	1	5	1	4	0	0	1	2
Lobster, boiled	34	119	0	0	1	3	0	0	6	22
Loganberries, fresh	5	17	1	3	0	0	2	6	0	1
Lorraine, quiche	65	230	5	17	4	15	0	0	2	8
Loganberries, stewed no sugar	5	16	1	3	0	0	2	6	0	1
Loganberries, tinned	29	101	7	26	0	0	1	3	0	1
Lucozade	19	68	5	18	0	0	0	0	0	0
Luncheon meat, tinned	87	304	2	7	7	25	1	2	4	13
Lychees	18	64	5	16	0	0	0	1	0	1

FOODS	Calories per		Carbohydrates per		Fat per		Fibre per		Protein per	
	oz	100g	oz	100g	oz	100g	oz	100g	oz	100g
Macaroni, raw short cut	94	332	20	72	1	2	1	3	3	11
Macaroni, cooked	44	156	10	34	0	1	1	2	2	6
Macaroni cheese	50	174	4	15	3	10	0	0	2	7
Macaroni cheese, tinned	34	118	4	13	2	6	0	0	1	5
Macaroons, coconut	113	397	18	62	5	16	2	6	1	5
Mackerel, fresh	52	182	0	0	4	12	0	0	5	18
Mackerel, kippered fillets	70	244	0	0	5	18	0	0	6	21
Mackerel, fried	54	188	0	0	3	11	0	0	6	22
Mackerel, smoked fresh	62	218	0	0	4	15	0	0	6	21
Madeira cake	112	393	18	60	6	20	1	1	2	5
Malt loaf	81	287	17	61	1	3	0	0	2	8
Malt vinegar	1	4	0	1	0	0	0	0	0	0
Malted milk [Horlicks] powder	112	396	21	73	2	8	0	0	4	14
Malted milk biscuits	135	472	20	71	5	19	0	0	2	8
Mandarin oranges, tinned	11	37	3	9	0	0	0	0	0	1
Mange Tout, cooked	10	34	2	6	0	0	0	0	1	3
Mango, raw	17	59	4	15	0	0	0	2	0	1
Mango, tinned	22	77	6	20	0	0	0	1	0	0
Margarine, all types	207	730	0	0	25	85	0	0	0	0
Marie biscuits	127	446	22	77	4	14	0	0	2	7

FOODS	Calories per oz	Calories per 100g	Carbohydrates per oz	per 100g	Fat per oz	per 100g	Fibre per oz	per 100g	Protein per oz	per 100g
Marmalade, all types average	72	253	19	67	0	0	0	1	0	0
Marmite	51	179	1	2	0	1	0	0	11	40
Marrow, boiled	2	7	0	1	0	0	1	1	0	0
Marzipan [almond paste]	127	443	14	49	7	25	2	6	2	9
Mayonnaise	208	734	0	0	23	81	0	0	1	2
Meats - see by name										
Meat pastes	49	173	1	3	3	11	0	0	4	15
Medlars	12	42	3	11	0	0	3	10	0	1
Melon, canteloupe fresh	7	24	2	5	0	0	1	1	0	1
Melon, honeydew fresh	6	21	1	5	0	0	1	1	0	1
Melon, water	6	21	2	5	0	0	1	1	0	0
Meringue	110	380	25	95	0	0	0	0	2	5
Milk, whole fresh	19	67	1	5	1	4	0	0	1	3
Milk, condensed sweetened	91	322	16	56	3	9	0	0	2	8
Milk, longlife UHT full cream	19	67	1	5	1	4	0	0	1	3
Milk, semi-skimmed fresh	14	48	1	5	1	2	0	0	1	3
Milk, skimmed dried	100	355	15	52	0	1	0	0	10	35
Milk, skimmed, fresh	9	34	1	5	0	0	0	0	1	3
Milk, skimmed UHT	10	34	1	5	0	0	0	0	1	4
Milk, condensed, skimmed sweetened	76	267	17	60	0	0	0	0	3	10

FOODS	Calories per oz	Calories per 100g	Carbohydrates per oz	Carbohydrates per 100g	Fat per oz	Fat per 100g	Fibre per oz	Fibre per 100g	Protein per oz	Protein per 100g
Milk, evaporated	44	154	3	11	3	9	0	0	2	8
Milk, dried	140	490	11	40	7	25	0	0	7	25
Milk, malted powder (Horlicks)	112	396	21	73	2	8	0	0	4	14
Milk pudding	37	131	6	20	1	4	0	0	1	4
Milk, soya	14	49	1	3	1	2	0	0	1	4
Milk, sterilised whole	19	67	1	5	1	4	0	0	1	3
Milk, sterilised skimmed	10	35	1	5	0	0	0	0	1	4
Milk, goats	20	71	1	5	1	5	0	0	1	3
Mincemeat	81	284	18	64	1	4	1	3	0	1
Mince pie	123	435	18	62	6	20	1	3	1	4
Minestrone soup, dried	87	305	19	65	1	2	1	3	3	11
Minestrone soup, tinned	9	33	2	6	0	1	0	0	0	1
Mint jelly	78	276	20	72	0	0	0	0	0	0
Mint sauce	5	18	1	5	0	0	0	0	0	1
Mints [Peppermints]	112	392	29	102	0	1	0	0	0	1
Mixed fruit, dried	71	247	18	64	0	0	2	7	1	2
Mixed peel	70	244	19	65	3	9	0	0	0	0
Mixed pepper	59	208	9	30	2	6	3	12	3	10
Mixed pickles	5	19	1	4	0	0	0	0	0	0
Mortadella	79	277	1	2	6	23	0	0	5	17

FOODS	Calories per oz	100g	Carbohydrates per oz	100g	Fat per oz	100g	Fibre per oz	100g	Protein per oz	100g
Moussaka	56	195	3	10	4	13	0	0	3	9
Mousse, flavoured frozen, average	47	163	7	23	2	7	0	0	1	4
Muesli, varies	93	330	18	63	2	6	3	11	3	10
Muffins	65	229	12	44	1	2	1	3	3	11
Muffins, Scottish	85	298	17	59	1	5	1	3	2	8
Muffins, wholemeal	61	215	11	39	1	3	2	7	3	10
Mulberries, raw	10	36	2	8	0	0	0	2	0	1
Mulligatawny soup, tinned	11	39	1	5	0	1	0	0	1	3
Mung beans, raw	66	231	10	36	0	1	6	22	6	22
Mung beans, cooked	46	161	8	28	0	0	1	5	4	13
Mung beans, cooked dahl	30	106	3	11	1	4	2	6	2	6
Mushroom quiche	73	257	6	20	5	17	0	1	2	8
Mushrooms raw, tinned or frozen	4	13	0	0	0	1	1	3	1	2
Mushrooms, fried	60	210	0	0	7	25	1	4	1	2
Mushrooms, sliced and dried	85	299	11	40	0	0	7	26	10	36
Mushroom soup, tinned	15	53	1	4	1	4	0	0	0	1
Mussels, fresh	16	56	0	0	1	2	0	0	3	10
Mustard powder, gross	130	450	6	20	8	30	0	0	8	30
Mustard, English	45	155	3	12	3	10	0	0	2	7
Mustard, French	21	75	1	4	1	4	0	0	2	6

FOODS	Calories per		Carbohydrates per		Fat per		Fibre per		Protein per	
	oz	100g	oz	100g	oz	100g	oz	100g	oz	100g
Mustard oil dressing	130	450	0	1	15	50	0	0	0	0
Mustard and cress, raw	3	10	0	1	0	0	1	4	0	2
Nectarines, fresh raw	14	50	4	12	0	0	1	2	0	1
Nice biscuits	130	456	21	75	5	16	0	0	2	7
Nutmeg, ground	129	456	8	30	10	35	0	0	2	8
Oatcakes	126	441	18	65	5	20	1	4	3	10
Oatmeal	115	401	21	73	2	9	2	7	4	12
Okra raw (Ladies fingers)	5	17	1	2	0	0	1	3	1	2
Olives in brine	29	103	0	0	3	11	1	4	0	1
Olives, cocktail pickle	31	111	1	5	3	10	0	0	0	1
Olive oil	251	887	0	0	30	100	0	0	0	0
Omelette, plain	54	190	0	0	5	16	0	0	3	11
Onion, raw	7	23	1	5	0	0	0	0	0	1
Onion bhajia	53	187	9	30	2	10	2	1	1	4
Onion, boiled	4	13	1	3	0	0	1	1	0	1

FOODS	Calories per		Carbohydrates per		Fat per		Fibre per		Protein per	
	oz	100g	oz	100g	oz	100g	oz	100g	oz	100g
Onions, cocktail pickle	3	10	1	2	0	0	0	0	0	1
Onion, dried, soup	75	262	16	56	0	1	2	6	3	11
Onion, fried	99	345	3	10	10	33	1	5	1	2
Onion, pickled	11	37	2	8	0	0	0	0	0	2
Onion spring, raw	10	35	2	9	0	0	1	3	0	1
Onion rings, fried	161	562	14	49	11	40	1	1	1	5
Onion sauce	31	110	4	15	1	4	0	0	1	5
Orange, fresh raw	10	35	2	9	0	0	1	2	0	1
Orange juice, fresh	12	43	3	11	0	0	0	0	0	1
Orange juice, tinned sweet	15	51	4	13	0	0	0	0	0	1
Orange juice, tinned unsweetened	9	33	2	9	0	0	0	0	0	0
Orange squash, high juice, undiluted	43	153	11	40	0	0	0	0	0	0
Orange whole drink, undiluted	27	95	7	25	0	0	0	0	0	0
Orangeade	7	23	2	6	0	0	0	0	0	0
Ovaltine, gross	108	378	23	81	1	4	0	0	3	10
Ox heart	51	180	0	0	2	6	0	0	9	32
Ox kidneys, stewed	49	172	0	0	2	8	0	0	7	26
Ox liver, stewed	56	198	1	4	3	10	0	0	7	25
Ox tongue, boiled	84	293	0	0	7	24	0	0	6	20
Oxo cubes, red	65	229	3	12	1	3	0	0	11	38

FOODS	Calories per oz	Calories per 100g	Carbohydrates per oz	Carbohydrates per 100g	Fat per oz	Fat per 100g	Fibre per oz	Fibre per 100g	Protein per oz	Protein per 100g
Oxtail, stewed	69	243	0	0	4	13	0	0	9	31
Oxtail soup, dried	95	333	18	62	1	3	1	3	5	18
Oxtail soup, tinned	10	36	2	6	0	1	0	0	1	2
Oysters, raw	14	51	0	0	0	1	0	0	3	11
Pale ale	9	32	1	2	0	0	0	0	0	0
Pancakes	87	307	10	36	5	16	0	1	2	6
Pancakes, potato	66	231	6	22	4	15	0	0	1	3
Pancakes, scotch	81	283	12	41	3	12	0	1	12	41
Pancake syrup	75	261	14	48	2	6	0	0	2	6
Papaya, tinned	19	65	5	17	0	0	0	1	0	0
Paprika	107	377	17	60	3	10	5	19	4	14
Parmesan cheese	139	492	0	0	10	36	0	0	12	44
Parsley, fresh	6	21	0	0	0	0	3	9	1	5
Parsley sauce mix	102	356	19	66	2	8	0	0	3	10
Parsley/thyme stuffing, made-up	25	86	5	18	0	1	0	0	1	2
Parsnips, boiled	24	86	5	18	0	1	0	0	0	2
Partridge, roast	60	212	0	0	2	7	0	0	10	40
Passion fruit	10	34	2	6	0	0	5	16	1	3
Pasta bows, shells, twists, uncooked	94	332	20	75	1	2	1	3	3	11

FOODS	Calories per oz	Calories per 100g	Carbohydrates per oz	Carbohydrates per 100g	Fat per oz	Fat per 100g	Fibre per oz	Fibre per 100g	Protein per oz	Protein per 100g
Pasty, Cornish	95	332	9	31	6	20	0	0	2	8
Pastrami	44	154	0	2	2	6	0	0	7	23
Pastry, choux cooked	94	330	9	31	6	20	0	1	2	9
Pastry, flaky cooked	161	565	14	47	12	41	1	2	2	6
Pastry, puff	114	398	10	37	8	26	0	2	2	6
Pastry, puff frozen	121	425	2	7	8	29	0	0	2	6
Pastry, shortcrust cooked	151	527	16	56	9	32	1	2	2	7
Pastry, shortcrust frozen	127	446	12	42	8	29	0	0	2	7
Pawpaw	13	45	3	11	0	0	0	0	0	1
Pea and ham soup, tinned	17	60	3	10	0	1	0	2	1	3
Peaches, fresh	10	37	3	9	0	0	0	1	0	1
Peaches, dried stewed no sugar	23	79	6	20	0	0	2	5	0	1
Peaches, tinned in juice	14	49	3	12	0	0	0	0	0	1
Peaches, tinned in syrup	19	68	5	18	0	0	0	0	0	0
Peanut butter	169	596	4	13	14	51	2	8	7	24
Peanuts, fresh or roasted	166	587	3	12	14	49	2	8	7	27
Peanuts and raisins	141	495	10	35	0	0	2	8	4	15
Pearl barley, boiled	30	105	6	22	0	1	1	2	1	4
Pearl barley, dried	102	360	24	84	0	2	2	7	2	8
Pears, avocado	64	223	1	2	6	22	1	2	1	4

FOODS	Calories per oz	100g	Carbohydrates per oz	100g	Fat per oz	100g	Fibre per oz	100g	Protein per oz	100g
Pears, fresh	8	29	2	8	0	0	1	2	0	0
Pears, stewed, no sugar	9	30	2	8	0	0	1	3	0	0
Pears, tinned in juice	15	54	4	13	0	0	0	1	0	0
Pears, tinned in syrup	20	69	5	18	0	0	0	1	0	0
Peas, chick cooked dahl	40	145	6	22	1	3	2	6	2	8
Peas, dried	81	286	14	50	0	1	5	17	6	22
Peas, fresh boiled	15	52	2	8	0	0	1	5	1	5
Peas, frozen	14	48	2	6	0	1	3	12	2	6
Peas, frozen boiled	12	41	1	4	0	0	3	12	2	5
Peas, garden tinned	13	47	2	7	0	0	2	6	1	5
Peas, marrow fat or processed	23	80	4	14	0	0	2	8	2	6
Peas, red pigeon raw	86	301	15	54	1	2	4	15	6	20
Pepper, black/white	87	308	20	68	2	7	0	0	3	9
Pepper, cayenne	114	402	16	58	4	14	5	16	4	14
Pepper, whole black	116	405	19	67	3	10	3	10	3	10
Pepper [chilli]	11	40	3	9	0	0	1	2	0	1
Peppers, green or red raw	4	15	1	2	0	0	0	1	0	1
Peppers, mixed frozen	5	16	1	2	0	0	0	0	0	1
Peppermint essence	86	301	0	0	0	0	0	0	0	0
Peppermints	112	392	30	102	0	1	0	0	0	1

FOODS	Calories per oz	100g	Carbohydrates per oz	100g	Fat per oz	100g	Fibre per oz	100g	Protein per oz	100g
Petit pois, frozen	15	53	2	7	0	1	2	8	1	5
Petit pois, tinned	23	82	5	16	0	0	1	3	1	5
Pheasant, roast	60	213	0	0	3	9	0	0	9	32
Piccalilli, sweet	24	84	6	21	0	0	0	1	0	1
Pigeon, roast	65	230	0	0	4	15	0	0	8	28
Pigeon peas	86	301	15	54	1	2	4	15	6	20
Pilchards in tomato sauce	36	126	0	1	2	5	0	0	5	19
Pineapple, fresh	13	46	3	12	0	5	0	1	0	1
Pineapple cubes, tinned in syrup	20	69	5	18	0	0	0	0	0	0
Pineapple jam	73	254	19	66	0	0	0	0	0	0
Pineapple, tinned in natural juice	15	52	4	13	0	0	0	1	0	1
Pineapple juice, tinned	15	53	4	13	0	0	0	0	0	0
Pineapple juice, longlife	11	39	3	10	0	0	0	5	0	0
Pinto beans	38	133	6	21	1	2	1	5	3	10
Pizza bread	74	258	17	60	0	1	2	9	2	6
PLJ pure lemon juice	2	7	0	2	0	0	0	0	0	0
Plaice fillet, fresh	25	86	0	0	0	2	0	0	5	18
Plaice fillet, frozen	26	91	0	0	1	2	0	0	5	18
Plaice, fried in batter	80	279	4	14	5	18	0	0	5	16
Plaice, fried in breadcrumbs	60	210	5	18	3	10	0	0	4	12

FOODS	Calories per oz	100g	Carbohydrates per oz	100g	Fat per oz	100g	Fibre per oz	100g	Protein per oz	100g
Plaice, steamed	27	93	0	0	1	2	0	0	5	19
Plantain, raw	32	112	8	28	0	0	2	6	0	1
Plantain, boiled	35	122	9	31	0	0	2	6	0	1
Plantain, fried	76	267	14	48	3	9	2	6	0	2
Plums, dessert raw	11	38	3	10	0	0	1	2	0	1
Plums, cooking raw	7	26	2	6	0	0	1	3	0	1
Plums, stewed no sugar	6	22	1	5	0	0	1	2	0	1
Plums, tinned in syrup	18	64	5	16	0	0	0	0	0	0
Plum jam	73	254	19	66	0	0	0	0	0	0
Plum pie	51	180	8	28	2	8	1	2	1	2
Polony sausage	80	281	4	14	6	21	0	0	3	9
Pomegranate	21	72	5	17	0	1	0	0	0	1
Pomegranate juice	13	44	3	12	0	0	0	0	0	0
Pork, chop grilled lean & fat	94	332	0	0	7	25	0	0	8	30
Pork, kidney stewed	43	153	0	0	2	6	0	0	7	24
Pork, roast leg, lean and fat	82	286	0	0	6	20	0	0	8	27
Pork, luncheon meat	87	304	2	7	7	25	1	2	4	13
Pork pate and mushrooms	98	344	2	6	9	32	0	0	3	9
Pork pie, Melton	107	376	6	21	8	29	0	0	3	9
Pork sausage, fried	91	317	3	10	7	25	0	0	4	15

FOODS	Calories per		Carbohydrates per		Fat per		Fibre per		Protein per	
	oz	100g	oz	100g	oz	100g	oz	100g	oz	100g
Pork sausage, grilled	91	318	3	12	7	25	0	0	4	13
Porridge, as served	12	44	2	8	0	1	0	1	0	1
Porridge oats, gross	108	382	19	68	2	9	2	7	4	12
Port wine	45	157	3	12	0	0	0	0	0	0
Potato, baked in jacket	31	107	7	25	0	0	1	3	1	3
Potato, boiled old	23	80	6	20	0	0	0	1	0	1
Potato, boiled new	22	77	5	18	0	0	1	2	0	2
Potato chips	72	253	11	37	3	11	0	0	1	4
Potato crisps	143	500	11	39	10	37	3	12	2	6
Potato croquettes, cooked	52	182	6	23	3	9	0	0	1	4
Potato instant mash, reconstituted	17	60	4	15	0	0	0	0	0	2
Potato, tinned	15	53	4	13	0	0	1	3	0	1
Potato salad	76	266	3	12	7	24	0	0	0	1
Potato salad with chives	54	190	5	17	4	14	0	1	0	1
Potato, sweet boiled	24	85	6	20	0	1	1	2	0	1
Prawn coleslaw	34	119	1	4	3	10	0	1	1	5
Prawn curry	28	99	5	16	1	2	0	0	1	4
Prawns, fresh	29	101	0	0	0	1	0	0	6	22
Prawn, frozen	28	98	0	0	0	1	0	0	6	22
Prawns, tinned	30	107	0	0	1	2	0	0	7	23

FOODS	Calories per		Carbohydrates per		Fat per		Fibre per		Protein per	
	oz	100g	oz	100g	oz	100g	oz	100g	oz	100g
Prawn salad	47	166	2	7	4	13	0	1	1	5
Processed cheese	89	313	0	0	8	30	0	0	4	14
Profiteroles	103	361	7	24	8	28	0	0	2	5
Profiteroles, frozen	106	372	5	19	9	32	0	0	1	4
Prunes, dried	46	161	12	40	0	0	5	16	1	2
Prunes, dried stewed no sugar	23	82	6	20	0	0	2	8	0	1
Prunes, tinned natural juice	33	117	9	31	0	0	1	5	0	1
Prunes, tinned in syrup	34	120	9	30	0	0	1	5	0	1
Puff pastry	114	398	10	37	8	26	0	2	2	6
Puff pastry, frozen	121	425	2	7	8	29	0	0	2	6
Puffed wheat	93	325	20	70	0	1	4	15	4	15
Pumpkin, boiled	6	21	1	5	0	0	0	1	0	1
Quiche, cauliflower fresh	70	246	5	19	5	16	1	2	2	7
Quiche, chicken asparagus	68	239	6	19	4	15	0	1	3	9
Quiche Lorraine	65	230	5	17	4	15	0	0	2	8
Quiche mushroom	73	257	6	20	5	17	0	1	2	8
Quince, fresh	7	25	2	6	0	0	2	6	0	0

FOODS	Calories per		Carbohydrates per		Fat per		Fibre per		Protein per	
	oz	100g	oz	100g	oz	100g	oz	100g	oz	100g
Rabbit, stewed	50	180	0	0	2	10	0	0	8	30
Radish, raw	4	15	1	3	0	0	0	1	0	1
Rainbow trout, frozen	39	135	0	0	2	7	0	0	5	19
Raisins, dried	70	246	18	64	0	0	2	7	0	1
Raspberries, fresh	7	25	2	6	0	0	2	7	0	1
Raspberries, tinned in natural juice	9	33	2	8	0	0	0	2	0	1
Raspberries, stewed no sugar	7	26	2	6	0	0	2	8	0	1
Raspberries, tinned in syrup	25	88	6	23	0	0	0	2	0	1
Raspberry jam	74	258	19	67	0	0	0	0	0	1
Raspberry gateau	55	194	8	27	3	9	1	2	1	4
Raspberry mousse, frozen	45	159	7	23	2	7	0	0	1	4
Raspberry ripple ice cream	47	164	7	25	2	6	0	0	1	3
Ratatouille, frozen	13	45	2	6	0	2	0	0	1	2
Ratatouille, tinned	13	46	1	4	1	3	0	1	0	1
Ravioli, tinned	23	80	4	14	1	2	0	1	1	2
Ready Brek	110	390	20	70	2	9	2	8	4	12
Red cabbage pickle	6	20	1	4	0	0	1	3	0	2
Redcurrants, raw	6	21	1	4	0	0	2	8	0	1
Redcurrants, stewed no sugar	5	18	1	4	0	0	2	7	0	1
Redcurrant jelly	73	256	19	67	0	0	0	0	0	0

FOODS	Calories per oz	Calories per 100g	Carbohydrates per oz	Carbohydrates per 100g	Fat per oz	Fat per 100g	Fibre per oz	Fibre per 100g	Protein per oz	Protein per 100g
Red kidney beans, cooked	29	101	5	17	0	1	3	9	2	8
Red Leicester cheese	114	398	0	0	10	34	0	0	7	24
Red mullet	35	122	0	0	1	5	0	0	5	19
Rhubarb, stewed no sugar	2	6	0	1	0	0	1	2	0	1
Rhubarb, tinned in syrup	16	56	4	14	0	0	0	2	0	1
Rhubarb custard, chilled	31	110	5	17	1	4	0	0	1	3
Rhubarb pie	51	180	8	28	2	8	1	2	1	2
Ribena, concentrated	65	229	17	61	0	0	0	0	0	0
Rice, boiled average	36	127	8	29	0	0	0	1	1	2
Rice, boil in bag	96	337	23	81	0	0	0	1	2	7
Rice, curried hot	31	109	7	25	0	1	0	1	1	2
Rice, curried mild	31	107	7	24	0	1	0	1	1	2
Rice, ground cooked	43	152	7	23	1	5	0	0	1	5
Rice Krispies	105	372	25	88	1	2	1	5	2	6
Rice pudding	43	152	5	19	2	7	0	1	1	5
Rice pudding, tinned creamed	25	88	5	16	0	2	0	0	1	3
Risotto, stir fry	21	75	5	16	0	1	1	3	1	3
Rock cakes	113	394	17	60	5	16	1	2	2	5
Rock salmon, fried in batter	76	265	2	8	5	19	0	0	5	17
Roe, cod hard fried	57	202	1	3	3	12	0	0	6	21

FOODS	Calories per		Carbohydrates per		Fat per		Fibre per		Protein per	
	oz	100g	oz	100g	oz	100g	oz	100g	oz	100g
Roe, herring soft fried	69	244	1	5	5	16	0	0	6	21
Rolls, brown crusty	83	289	16	57	1	3	2	6	3	12
Rolls, brown soft	81	282	14	48	2	6	2	5	3	12
Rolls, white crusty	83	290	16	57	1	3	1	3	3	12
Rolls white soft	87	305	15	54	2	7	1	3	3	10
Roquefort cheese	101	355	0	0	8	30	0	0	7	25
Rosehip syrup, neat	66	232	18	62	0	0	0	0	0	0
Rye flour	96	335	22	76	1	2	0	0	2	8
Ryvita crispbread	92	321	20	71	1	2	3	12	3	9
Sage and onion stuffing, made-up	32	112	7	23	0	1	0	0	1	3
Sago pudding	39	136	5	18	2	6	0	0	1	4
St Paulin cheese	86	305	0	0	7	23	0	0	7	25
Saithe [coalfish] steamed	28	99	0	0	0	1	0	0	7	23
Salad cream	92	324	5	18	8	28	0	1	0	1
Salami, average	140	490	1	2	13	45	0	0	6	20
Salmon, smoked Scottish	48	170	0	0	3	10	0	0	6	20
Salmon, steaks frozen	52	181	0	0	3	12	0	0	5	18
Salmon, steamed	56	197	0	0	4	13	0	0	6	20
Salmon, pink tinned	40	141	0	0	1	5	0	0	6	20

FOODS	Calories per oz	Calories per 100g	Carbohydrates per oz	Carbohydrates per 100g	Fat per oz	Fat per 100g	Fibre per oz	Fibre per 100g	Protein per oz	Protein per 100g
Salmon, red tinned	44	153	0	0	2	8	0	0	6	20
Salmon spread	40	140	0	1	2	8	0	0	5	17
Salmon and shrimp paste	52	183	1	2	0	0	0	0	5	17
Salsisfy, boiled	5	18	1	3	0	0	0	0	1	2
Salt, cooking and table	0	0	0	0	0	0	0	0	0	0
Sandwich spread	58	203	7	26	3	11	0	0	0	2
Sardine and tomato paste	53	185	1	3	3	12	0	0	5	18
Sardines, tinned in oil	95	334	0	0	8	28	0	0	6	20
Sardines in tomato sauce	51	177	0	1	3	12	0	0	5	18
Satsumas, fresh	10	34	2	8	0	0	1	2	0	1
Sauce Tartare	77	271	5	18	6	22	0	0	1	2
Sausage, beef fried	76	269	4	15	5	18	0	0	4	13
Sausage, beef grilled	75	265	4	15	5	17	0	0	4	13
Sausage, cocktail	91	319	4	13	7	25	0	0	4	12
Sausage, liver	65	230	2	8	5	17	0	0	4	13
Sausage, pork fried	91	317	3	11	7	25	0	0	4	14
Sausage, pork grilled	91	318	3	12	7	25	0	0	4	13
Sausage roll, flaky pastry	137	479	9	33	10	36	0	0	2	7
Sausage, chipolatas	81	285	3	10	6	22	0	0	4	13
Sausage, frankfurters	78	274	1	3	7	25	0	0	3	10

FOODS	Calories per oz	Calories per 100g	Carbohydrates per oz	Carbohydrates per 100g	Fat per oz	Fat per 100g	Fibre per oz	Fibre per 100g	Protein per oz	Protein per 100g
Sausage, saveloy	74	262	3	10	6	21	0	0	3	10
Sauternes wine	27	94	2	6	0	0	0	0	0	0
Scallops, steamed	30	105	0	0	0	1	0	0	7	23
Scampi, fried in breadcrumbs	90	316	8	29	5	18	0	0	3	12
Scones	106	371	16	56	4	15	1	2	2	8
Scones, soda	77	269	13	45	2	8	0	0	2	8
Scotch broth soup, tinned	11	40	2	7	0	1	0	0	0	2
Scotch egg	80	279	3	12	6	20	0	0	3	10
Scotch pancakes	81	283	12	41	3	12	1	1	2	7
Seakale, boiled	2	8	0	1	0	0	1	1	0	1
Semolina, cooked	43	151	6	22	1	5	0	0	2	6
Semolina, packet	100	350	22	78	1	2	0	0	3	11
Shallot, raw	14	48	3	10	0	0	0	0	1	2
Shepherds pie, frozen	35	123	3	11	2	7	0	0	1	5
Sherry, dry	33	116	0	1	0	0	0	0	0	0
Sherry, medium	34	118	1	4	0	0	0	0	0	0
Sherry, sweet	39	136	2	7	0	0	0	0	0	0
Shortbread biscuits (shortcake)	149	523	17	61	9	30	1	2	2	6
Shortcrust pastry, cooked	151	527	16	56	9	32	1	2	2	7
Shortcrust pastry, frozen	127	446	12	42	8	29	0	0	2	7

FOODS	Calories per		Carbohydrates per		Fat per		Fibre per		Protein per	
	oz	100g	oz	100g	oz	100g	oz	100g	oz	100g
Shredded Wheat	92	324	19	68	1	3	3	12	3	11
Shrimps, fresh	22	77	0	0	0	1	0	0	5	17
Shrimps, tinned	27	94	0	0	0	1	0	0	6	21
Skate, fresh	27	94	0	0	0	1	0	0	6	21
Skate, fried in batter	57	199	1	5	3	12	0	0	5	18
Skimmed milk, dried	100	355	15	55	0	1	0	0	10	35
Skimmed milk, fresh	9	34	1	5	0	0	0	0	1	3
Smoked haddock mousse paté	78	273	0	1	7	26	0	0	3	11
Smoked mackerel, fresh	62	218	0	0	4	15	0	0	6	21
Smoked mackerel, frozen	86	302	0	0	7	25	0	0	6	20
Smoked salmon, fresh	48	170	0	0	3	10	0	0	6	20
Smoked salmon paté	83	292	0	1	7	25	0	0	5	17
Smoked trout	74	259	0	0	6	22	0	0	5	16
Smoked trout pate	73	259	0	0	6	22	0	0	5	16
Smoked turkey paté	101	354	0	1	10	35	0	0	3	11
Soda bread	75	264	16	56	1	2	1	2	2	8
Soda water	0	0	0	0	0	0	0	0	0	0
Sole, dover fresh	23	81	0	0	0	1	0	0	5	18
Sole, dover or lemon fried	61	216	3	9	4	13	0	0	5	16
Sole, dover or lemon steamed	26	90	0	0	0	1	0	0	6	20

FOODS	Calories per		Carbohydrates per		Fat per		Fibre per		Protein per	
	oz	100g	oz	100g	oz	100g	oz	100g	oz	100g
Soufflé cheese	70	250	3	9	5	20	0	0	3	12
Southern stir fry	16	55	3	10	0	1	1	4	1	3
Soya flour, full fat	128	447	7	24	7	24	3	12	11	37
Soya flour, low fat	101	352	8	28	2	7	4	14	13	45
Soya oil	255	900	0	0	30	100	0	0	0	0
Spaghetti, raw	94	332	20	72	1	2	1	3	3	11
Spaghetti, boiled	38	134	8	29	0	0	0	2	2	5
Spaghetti bolognaise mix	83	290	19	67	0	0	0	0	3	11
Spaghetti in tomato sauce	17	59	3	12	0	1	0	0	0	2
Spaghetti, verdi cooked	37	130	8	29	0	0	0	2	1	4
Special K cereal	110	388	22	78	1	3	2	6	5	18
Spice, mixed	105	367	19	65	3	10	7	25	2	8
Spinach, boiled	9	30	0	1	0	1	2	6	1	5
Spinach leaf frozen	9	31	1	5	0	0	2	6	1	3
Spirits 70% proof, neat	65	225	0	0	0	0	0	0	0	0
Sponge cake, no fat	86	301	15	54	2	7	0	1	3	10
Sponge cake, with fat	133	464	15	53	5	20	0	1	2	6
Sponge fingers	110	384	25	86	1	3	0	0	2	7
Sponge flan case	85	299	19	65	1	3	0	0	2	6
Sponge cake, jam	86	302	18	64	1	5	0	1	1	4

FOODS	Calories per oz	100g	Carbohydrates per oz	100g	Fat per oz	100g	Fibre per oz	100g	Protein per oz	100g
Sponge pudding, jam	97	341	17	59	3	11	0	0	1	4
Sponge trifle	87	305	20	70	1	2	0	0	1	5
Spotted dick	91	320	17	59	3	9	0	0	1	4
Sprats, fresh	40	139	0	0	3	9	0	0	4	15
Sprats, gross fried	126	441	0	0	11	38	0	0	7	25
Spring greens, boiled	3	12	0	1	0	0	1	4	0	2
Spring onions	10	35	2	9	0	0	1	3	0	1
Sprouts brussels, boiled	5	18	0	2	0	0	0	0	1	3
Squid	23	80	0	0	0	1	0	0	5	17
Steak, beef rump fried	70	246	0	0	4	15	0	0	8	29
Steak, grilled lean/fat	62	218	0	0	3	12	0	0	8	27
Steak, stewing stewed	64	220	0	0	3	11	0	0	9	30
Steak, stewed tinned	41	142	1	2	2	8	0	1	4	15
Steaks, grill	86	301	0	1	7	26	1	1	5	16
Steak & kidney pie	71	250	6	20	4	15	0	0	3	9
Steak and kidney pie, frozen	92	254	6	23	4	15	0	0	3	10
Steak and kidney pudding	49	171	3	11	3	10	0	0	3	11
Stilton cheese	132	462	0	0	11	40	0	0	7	26
Stout, bottled	10	37	1	4	0	0	0	0	0	0
Stout, strong bottled	11	39	1	2	0	0	0	0	0	0

FOODS	Calories per		Carbohydrates per		Fat per		Fibre per		Protein per	
	oz	100g	oz	100g	oz	100g	oz	100g	oz	100g
Strawberries, fresh	7	26	2	6	0	0	1	2	0	1
Strawberries, tinned in natural juice	10	36	3	9	0	0	0	1	0	1
Strawberries, tinned in syrup	21	75	5	19	0	0	0	1	0	1
Strawberry jam	73	257	19	67	0	0	0	0	0	0
Strawberry mousse, frozen	45	159	7	23	2	7	0	0	1	4
Strawberry pie filling, tinned	20	70	5	18	0	0	0	0	0	0
Strong ale	21	70	2	6	0	0	0	0	0	1
Stuffing, Country herb, made up	31	109	6	22	0	1	0	0	1	3
Stuffing, parsley and thyme, made up	25	86	5	18	0	1	0	0	1	2
Stuffing, sage and onion, made up	32	112	7	23	0	1	0	0	1	3
Suet, butchers block	254	895	0	0	30	100	0	0	0	1
Suet, shredded beef	230	813	3	12	25	85	0	0	0	0
Suet pudding, with syrup	92	323	17	59	3	10	0	0	1	3
Sugar	108	382	28	100	0	0	0	0	0	0
Sugar Puffs	99	348	24	85	0	1	2	6	2	6
Sultanas, dried	89	312	22	79	0	0	2	7	1	3
Sunflower oil	255	900	0	0	30	100	0	0	0	0
Swede, boiled	5	18	1	4	0	0	1	3	0	1
Sweet and sour chicken, tinned	25	88	2	8	1	3	0	0	2	8
Sweet and sour sauce	93	325	21	73	1	4	0	0	1	4

FOODS	Calories per		Carbohydrates per		Fat per		Fibre per		Protein per	
	oz	100g	oz	100g	oz	100g	oz	100g	oz	100g
Sweet pickles	39	136	10	35	0	0	0	0	0	1
Sweetbreads lamb, fried	65	230	2	6	4	15	0	0	5	19
Sweetcorn, tinned	21	75	5	16	0	0	2	6	1	3
Sweet potato, cooked	24	85	6	20	0	1	1	2	0	1
Swiss roll, chocolate	113	396	15	52	6	21	0	0	1	3
Swiss roll, strawberry	105	366	17	59	4	15	0	0	1	2
Swordfish	33	117	0	0	1	4	0	0	5	19
Syrup, golden	85	298	23	79	0	0	0	0	0	0
Syrup pudding	92	323	17	59	3	10	0	0	1	3
Tagliatelle, cooked	38	134	8	29	0	0	0	2	2	5
Tangerines, fresh	10	34	2	8	0	0	1	2	0	1
Tapioca, cooked	35	121	5	19	1	4	0	0	2	6
Tapioca, seed pearl	102	359	27	95	0	0	0	0	0	0
Taramasalata	118	413	2	8	12	41	0	0	1	4
Tart custard	82	287	8	30	5	17	0	1	2	6
Tart, jam	110	384	18	63	4	15	0	2	1	4
Tart, treacle	105	371	18	61	4	14	0	1	1	4
Tartare sauce	77	271	5	18	6	22	0	0	1	2
Tea, black all types, infusion	0	0	0	0	0	0	0	0	0	0

FOODS	Calories per		Carbohydrates per		Fat per		Fibre per		Protein per	
	oz	100g	oz	100g	oz	100g	oz	100g	oz	100g
Tea cake	77	270	16	57	1	4	0	0	1	5
Thousand Island dressing	77	273	3	9	7	25	0	0	1	2
Toast, white	85	297	19	65	1	2	1	3	3	10
Tomato, fresh raw	4	14	1	3	0	0	0	2	0	1
Tomato, fried	20	69	1	3	2	6	1	3	0	1
Tomato, tinned	5	16	1	3	0	0	0	0	0	1
Tomato chutney	44	154	11	40	0	0	1	2	0	1
Tomato juice, tinned	5	16	1	3	0	0	0	0	0	1
Tomato ketchup, average	35	123	9	29	0	1	0	0	0	1
Tomato paste	25	87	5	19	0	0	0	1	1	3
Tomato puree	19	67	3	11	0	0	0	0	2	6
Tomato relish	34	120	9	30	0	0	0	0	0	1
Tomato sauce	24	86	2	8	1	5	1	2	1	2
Tomato, cheese, pineapple ham pizza	57	198	9	30	2	5	2	2	3	10
Tomato soup, creamed tinned	22	77	3	11	1	4	0	0	0	1
Tongue, lamb tinned	61	213	0	0	5	17	0	0	5	16
Tongue, ox boiled	84	293	0	0	7	24	0	0	6	20
Tongue, sheep stewed	82	289	0	0	7	24	0	0	5	18
Tonic water	8	28	2	8	0	0	0	0	0	0
Treacle, black	73	257	19	67	0	0	0	0	1	1

FOODS	Calories per oz	Calories per 100g	Carbohydrates per oz	Carbohydrates per 100g	Fat per oz	Fat per 100g	Fibre per oz	Fibre per 100g	Protein per oz	Protein per 100g
Treacle tart	105	371	18	60	4	15	0	1	1	4
Trifle, fruit as served	43	149	5	18	2	8	0	0	1	2
Trifle sponge	87	305	20	70	1	2	0	0	1	5
Tripe, dressed	17	60	0	0	1	3	0	0	3	9
Tripe, stewed	28	100	0	0	1	5	0	0	4	15
Trout fillet, steamed	39	135	0	0	1	5	0	0	7	24
Trout, fresh	39	135	0	0	2	7	0	0	5	19
Tuna fish in oil	64	227	0	0	5	17	0	0	6	21
Tuna mayonnaise paste	67	236	0	1	5	17	0	0	5	17
Tuna paté	108	379	0	0	10	36	0	0	4	15
Turkey breast, roast	29	103	0	0	0	1	0	0	7	23
Turkey leg, roast	42	148	0	0	1	4	0	0	8	28
Turkey, roast with skin	48	171	0	0	2	7	0	0	8	28
Turnips, boiled	4	14	1	2	0	1	1	2	0	1
Ugli fruit	14	50	3	12	0	0	0	0	0	1

FOODS	Calories per		Carbohydrates per		Fat per		Fibre per		Protein per	
	oz	100g	oz	100g	oz	100g	oz	100g	oz	100g
Vanilla essence	67	236	0	0	0	0	0	0	0	0
Veal cutlet, fried	61	215	1	4	2	8	0	0	9	31
Veal, jellied tinned	36	125	0	0	1	3	0	0	7	25
Veal, roast	66	230	0	0	3	12	0	0	9	32
Vegetable oils	255	900	0	0	30	100	0	0	0	0
Vegetable paté	30	106	2	8	2	5	1	3	2	7
Vegetable pizza, chilled	63	219	8	28	3	8	0	0	3	9
Vegetable salad	59	208	4	14	5	17	0	2	0	2
Vegetable soup	14	51	3	9	0	1	0	0	1	2
Vegetable stock cubes	84	295	5	18	6	20	0	0	4	15
Venison, roast	56	198	0	0	2	6	0	0	10	35
Vermicelli	30	104	6	22	0	1	0	1	1	4
Vermouth, dry	34	118	2	6	0	0	0	0	0	0
Vermouth, sweet	43	151	5	16	0	0	0	0	0	0
Vinegar, cider	1	3	0	1	0	0	0	0	0	0
Vinegar, distilled	1	4	0	1	0	0	0	0	0	0
Vinegar, malt	1	4	0	1	0	0	0	0	0	0

FOODS	Calories per oz	Calories per 100g	Carbohydrates per oz	Carbohydrates per 100g	Fat per oz	Fat per 100g	Fibre per oz	Fibre per 100g	Protein per oz	Protein per 100g
Wafer filled biscuits	153	535	19	66	9	30	1	2	1	5
Walnuts, shelled	150	525	1	5	15	52	1	5	3	11
Water biscuits	113	396	21	73	3	9	1	3	3	10
Watercress, fresh	4	14	0	1	0	0	1	3	1	3
Watermelon	621	2	5	0	0	0	1	0	0	
Weetabix/Weetaflakes	96	340	20	70	1	3	4	13	3	11
Welsh rarebit	103	365	7	24	7	24	0	0	4	16
Wensleydale cheese	107	375	0	0	9	31	0	0	7	23
Wheatgerm bread	69	243	13	46	1	3	1	5	3	10
Whelks, fresh or boiled	26	92	0	0	1	2	0	0	5	19
Whipping cream	103	364	1	3	11	39	0	0	1	2
Whisky neat 70% proof	63	222	0	0	0	0	0	0	0	0
White currants, raw	7	26	2	6	0	0	2	7	0	1
White currants, stewed no sugar	6	22	1	5	0	0	2	6	0	1
White fish fillets, frozen	23	80	0	0	0	1	0	0	5	18
White sauce, savoury	43	151	3	11	3	10	0	0	1	4
White sauce, sweet	49	172	5	19	3	10	0	0	1	4
Whitebait, fried	150	525	2	5	15	50	0	0	6	20
Whiting, fresh	22	78	0	0	0	1	0	0	5	18
Whiting, fried	55	191	2	7	3	10	0	0	5	18

FOODS	Calories per		Carbohydrates per		Fat per		Fibre per		Protein per	
	oz	100g	oz	100g	oz	100g	oz	100g	oz	100g
Whiting, steamed	26	92	0	0	0	1	0	0	6	21
Whole lemon drink, undiluted	29	103	8	27	0	0	0	0	0	0
Whole orange drink, undiluted	27	95	7	25	0	0	0	0	0	0
Wholemeal bran biscuits	125	439	17	60	6	20	2	7	2	8
Wholemeal bread	69	242	14	48	1	2	2	9	3	10
Wholemeal flour, stoneground	90	318	20	70	1	2	3	10	4	15
Wine, red	19	68	0	0	0	0	0	0	0	0
Wine, rose	20	71	1	3	0	0	0	0	0	0
Wine, white dry	19	66	0	1	0	0	0	0	0	0
Wine, white medium	21	75	1	3	0	0	0	0	0	0
Wine, white sweet	27	94	2	6	0	0	0	0	0	0
Wine sauce, red	13	47	2	6	0	2	0	0	0	1
Wine sauce, white	21	74	2	6	1	5	0	0	0	1
Wine, sparkling white	22	76	0	1	0	0	0	0	0	0
Winkles, boiled	21	74	0	0	0	1	0	0	4	15
Worcestershire sauce	32	112	8	27	0	1	0	0	0	1

FOODS	Calories per oz	100g	Carbohydrates per oz	100g	Fat per oz	100g	Fibre per oz	100g	Protein per oz	100g
Yam, boiled	34	119	9	30	0	0	1	4	0	2
Yeast, dried	48	169	1	4	0	2	6	22	10	36
Yellow split peas, cooked	39	137	7	24	0	1	1	5	3	11
Yoghourt, natural	15	52	2	6	0	1	0	0	1	5
Yoghourt, flavoured	23	81	4	15	0	1	0	0	1	5
Yoghourt, fruit	27	95	5	18	0	1	0	0	1	5
Yoghourt, apple	23	80	4	14	0	1	0	0	1	5
Yoghourt, apricot	27	95	5	18	0	1	0	0	1	5
Yoghourt, blackcurrant	27	96	5	19	0	1	0	0	1	5
Yoghourt, chocolate	27	94	5	17	0	1	0	0	1	5
Yoghourt, hazelnut	30	106	5	17	1	3	0	0	1	5
Yoghourt, strawberry	25	89	5	17	0	1	0	0	1	5
Yorkshire pudding	61	215	7	25	3	10	0	1	2	7

Section 2

Food listings by variety & type

FOODS	Calories per		Carbohydrates per		Fat per		Fibre per		Protein per	
	oz	100g	oz	100g	oz	100g	oz	100g	oz	100g
BEVERAGES										
Bournvita gross	108	377	23	79	1	5	0	0	2	9
Bovril meat extract gross	50	174	1	3	0	1	0	0	11	38
Chocolate drinking powder made up	28	99	3	12	1	4	0	0	1	4
Chocolate drinking gross	106	374	23	80	2	6	0	0	1	5
Cocoa	91	317	3	12	6	22	0	0	6	20
Coffee black	0	0	0	0	0	0	0	0	0	0
Coffee instant gross	30	100	3	10	0	0	0	0	4	15
Horlicks malted milk gross	112	396	21	73	2	10	0	0	4	15
Marmite gross	51	179	1	2	0	1	0	0	11	40
Ovaltine gross	108	378	23	81	1	4	0	0	3	10
Ribena concentrated	65	229	17	61	0	0	0	0	0	0
Tea black all types, infusion	0	0	0	0	0	0	0	0	0	0
BISCUITS										
Cheese biscuits	143	505	15	53	8	30	0	0	3	10
Chocolate all over	150	524	20	65	8	28	1	3	2	6
Cream crackers	125	440	20	68	5	16	1	3	3	10
Digestive chocolate	141	493	20	65	8	25	1	3	2	7
Digestive plain	135	471	19	66	6	20	2	5	3	10
Figroll	97	338	20	69	2	6	2	7	1	4
Garibaldi	111	390	22	77	3	9	0	0	1	4
Ginger nuts	130	456	25	80	4	15	1	2	2	6

FOODS	Calories per oz	Calories per 100g	Carbohydrates per oz	Carbohydrates per 100g	Fat per oz	Fat per 100g	Fibre per oz	Fibre per 100g	Protein per oz	Protein per 100g
Lincoln	138	482	20	70	6	21	0	0	2	7
Malted milk	135	472	20	71	5	19	0	0	2	8
Marie	127	446	22	77	4	14	0	0	2	7
Nice	130	456	21	75	5	16	0	0	2	7
Shortbread (shortcake)	149	523	17	61	9	30	0	0	2	6
Wafer filled	153	535	19	66	9	30	1	2	1	5
Water	113	396	21	73	3	9	1	3	3	10
Wholemeal bran	125	439	17	60	6	20	2	7	2	8
BREAD										
Baguettes, frozen	73	255	16	57	0	1	1	3	2	7
Bread brown	71	249	13	52	1	2	1	5	2	8
Bread Hovis	69	243	13	46	1	3	1	5	3	10
Bread garlic white	117	409	14	47	6	22	1	2	2	8
Bread white [1 thin slice = 1 oz]	67	233	14	50	1	2	1	3	2	8
Bread wholemeal	69	242	14	48	1	2	2	9	3	10
Bread white fried	159	558	15	51	11	37	1	2	3	8
Bread white toasted	85	297	19	65	1	2	1	3	3	10
Bread rolls crusty brown	85	290	15	55	1	3	2	6	3	12
Bread rolls crusty white	85	290	15	55	1	3	1	3	3	12
Bread rolls soft brown	81	282	14	48	2	6	2	5	3	12
Bread rolls soft white	87	305	15	54	2	7	1	3	3	10
Bread currant	71	250	15	52	1	3	1	2	2	6

FOODS	Calories per oz	Calories per 100g	Carbohydrates per oz	Carbohydrates per 100g	Fat per oz	Fat per 100g	Fibre per oz	Fibre per 100g	Protein per oz	Protein per 100g
Bread soda	75	264	16	56	1	2	1	2	2	8
Crispbread rye	92	321	20	71	1	2	3	12	3	9
Crispbread wheat	110	390	10	40	2	8	1	5	15	45
Croissants	121	424	13	46	7	24	0	0	3	9
Crumpets	49	170	11	37	0	0	1	2	2	7
Malt loaf	81	287	17	61	1	3	0	0	2	8
Muffins	65	229	12	44	1	2	1	3	3	11
Muffins scottish	85	298	17	59	1	5	1	3	2	8
Muffins wholemeal	61	215	11	39	1	3	2	7	3	10
BREAKFAST CEREALS										
All-Bran	77	273	12	43	2	6	8	27	4	15
Bemax gross	99	347	13	45	2	8	0	0	8	26
Bran Flakes	94	329	20	72	1	2	4	15	3	9
Bran wheat	59	206	8	27	2	6	13	44	4	14
Cornflakes	105	370	25	85	0	2	3	10	2	10
Grapenuts	100	355	22	75	1	3	2	7	3	10
Muesli unsweetened	93	330	18	63	2	6	3	11	3	10
Porridge oats gross	108	382	19	68	2	9	2	7	4	12
Porridge as served	12	44	2	8	0	1	0	1	0	1
Puffed Wheat	93	325	20	70	0	1	4	15	4	15
Ready Brek	110	390	20	70	2	9	2	8	4	12
Rice Krispies	105	372	25	88	1	2	1	5	2	6

FOODS	Calories per		Carbohydrates per		Fat per		Fibre per		Protein per	
	oz	100g	oz	100g	oz	100g	oz	100g	oz	100g
Shredded Wheat	92	324	19	68	1	3	3	12	3	11
Special K	110	388	22	78	1	3	2	6	5	18
Sugar Puffs	99	348	24	85	0	1	2	6	2	6
Weetabix/Weetaflakes	96	340	20	70	1	3	4	13	3	11
CAKES										
Coconut slice	100	351	20	71	2	8	0	0	1	3
Fancy iced	116	407	19	67	4	15	1	2	1	4
Fruit plain	100	354	17	58	4	13	1	3	1	5
Fruit iced	100	352	18	62	4	13	1	3	1	4
Fruit rich	95	337	17	58	4	13	1	3	1	4
Gingerbread	107	373	18	63	4	13	0	1	2	6
Madeira	112	393	18	60	6	20	1	1	2	5
Mince pies	123	435	18	62	6	20	1	3	1	4
Rock	113	394	17	60	5	16	1	2	2	5
Sponge [no fat]	86	301	15	54	2	7	0	1	3	10
Sponge [with fat]	133	464	15	53	5	20	0	1	2	6
Sponge, jam	86	302	18	64	1	5	0	1	1	4
Swiss roll, chocolate	113	396	15	52	6	21	0	0	1	3
Swiss roll, strawberry	105	366	17	59	4	15	0	0	1	2
Teacake	77	270	16	57	1	4	0	0	1	5
Trifle sponge	87	305	20	70	1	2	0	0	1	5

FOODS	Calories per		Carbohydrates per		Fat per		Fibre per		Protein per	
	oz	100g	oz	100g	oz	100g	oz	100g	oz	100g
CHEESE (*see Dairy Products*)										
CHEESE DISHES										
Cauliflower cheese	29	100	2	8	2	6	0	1	2	6
Cheese, macaroni	50	174	4	15	3	10	0	0	2	7
Cheese pudding	48	170	2	8	3	11	0	0	3	10
Cheese soufflé	70	250	3	9	5	20	0	0	3	12
Cheese and tomato pizza	75	262	10	36	2	8	0	0	4	13
Quiche Lorraine	65	230	5	17	4	15	0	0	2	8
Welsh rarebit	103	365	7	24	7	24	0	0	4	16
CONDIMENTS (*see also Salad Dressings*)										
Apple sauce	27	94	7	24	0	0	0	0	0	0
Cinnamon	95	337	23	80	1	2	6	20	1	5
Cloves	118	413	20	69	4	15	3	11	2	6
Cranberry sauce	39	137	10	36	0	0	0	0	0	0
Curry powder	66	233	7	26	3	11	0	0	3	10
Horseradish sauce	53	185	5	18	3	11	1	2	1	3
Mint jelly	78	276	20	72	0	0	0	0	0	0
Mint sauce	5	18	1	5	0	0	0	0	0	1
Mustard, English	45	155	3	12	3	10	0	0	2	7
Mustard, French	21	75	1	4	1	4	0	0	2	6

FOODS	Calories per		Carbohydrates per		Fat per		Fibre per		Protein per	
	oz	100g	oz	100g	oz	100g	oz	100g	oz	100g
Mustard powder	130	450	6	20	8	30	0	0	8	30
Nutmeg whole	158	556	23	80	1	2	1	3	2	7
Nutmeg ground	129	456	8	30	10	35	0	0	2	8
Paprika	107	377	17	60	3	10	5	19	4	14
Pepper black/white	87	308	20	68	2	7	5	0	3	9
Pepper cayenne	114	402	16	58	4	14	5	16	4	14
Redcurrant jelly	73	256	19	67	0	0	0	0	0	0
Salt cooking and table	0	0	0	0	0	0	0	0	0	0
Sauce tartare	77	271	5	18	6	22	0	0	1	2
Spice mixed	105	367	19	65	3	10	7	25	2	8
DAIRY PRODUCTS										
Cheese										
Brie	89	310	0	0	7	24	0	0	6	20
Caerphilly	105	367	0	0	9	30	0	0	7	23
Camembert	82	289	0	0	7	24	0	0	5	19
Cheddar	115	406	0	0	10	34	0	0	7	26
Cheshire	106	371	0	0	9	31	0	0	7	24
Cottage cheese	28	98	1	3	1	4	0	0	4	13
Cream cheese	125	440	0	0	15	50	0	0	1	3
Danish blue	97	342	0	0	8	30	0	0	5	20
Edam	86	305	0	0	7	23	0	0	7	25
Emmental	138	486	0	0	8	30	0	0	8	30

FOODS	Calories per oz	Calories per 100g	Carbohydrates per oz	Carbohydrates per 100g	Fat per oz	Fat per 100g	Fibre per oz	Fibre per 100g	Protein per oz	Protein per 100g
Gorgonzola	101	355	0	0	8	29	0	0	7	23
Gouda	87	305	0	0	7	23	0	0	7	25
Gruyere	126	446	0	0	9	33	0	0	11	38
Parmesan	139	492	0	0	10	36	0	0	12	44
Processed cheese	89	313	0	0	8	30	0	0	4	14
Roquefort	101	355	0	0	8	30	0	0	7	25
St Paulin	86	305	0	0	7	23	0	0	7	25
Stilton	132	462	0	0	11	40	0	0	7	26
Wensleydale	107	375	0	0	9	31	0	0	7	23
Cream										
Cream clotted	156	550	0	1	17	60	0	0	0	1
Cream double	128	447	1	2	15	50	0	0	0	2
Cream single	55	193	1	4	5	19	0	0	1	3
Cream soured	54	190	1	3	5	18	0	0	1	3
Cream tinned sterilised	68	240	1	4	7	25	0	0	1	3
Cream whipping	103	364	1	3	11	39	0	0	1	2
Eggs										
Eggs, raw or boiled	42	148	0	0	3	10	0	0	3	12
Eggs, dried gross	161	564	0	0	12	45	0	0	12	45
Eggs, fried	66	232	0	0	6	20	0	0	4	15
Eggs, omelette	54	190	0	0	5	15	0	0	3	10

FOODS	Calories per		Carbohydrates per		Fat per		Fibre per		Protein per	
	oz	100g	oz	100g	oz	100g	oz	100g	oz	100g
Eggs, scotch	80	279	3	12	6	20	0	0	3	10
Eggs, scrambled	70	246	0	0	6	20	0	0	3	10
Eggs, white raw	10	36	0	0	0	0	0	0	3	10
Eggs, yolk raw	95	340	0	0	9	30	0	0	5	16
Milk										
Channel Island	22	76	1	5	1	5	0	0	1	4
Condensed sweetened	91	322	16	56	3	9	0	0	2	8
Condensed skimmed sweetened	76	267	17	60	0	0	0	0	3	10
Dried	140	490	11	40	7	25	0	0	7	25
Dried skimmed	100	355	15	52	0	1	0	0	10	35
Evaporated	44	154	3	11	3	9	0	0	2	8
Goats	20	71	1	5	1	5	0	0	1	3
Malted	110	385	21	72	2	7	0	0	4	13
Semi-skimmed fresh	14	48	1	5	1	2	0	0	1	3
Skimmed fresh	9	34	1	5	0	0	0	0	1	3
Skimmed dried	100	355	15	52	0	1	0	0	10	35
Skimmed UHT	10	34	1	5	0	0	0	0	1	4
Soya	14	49	1	3	1	2	0	0	1	4
Sterilised skimmed	10	35	1	5	0	0	0	0	1	4
Sterilised whole & UHT	19	67	1	5	1	4	0	0	1	3
Whole fresh	19	67	1	5	1	4	0	0	1	3

FOODS	Calories per oz	100g	Carbohydrates per oz	100g	Fat per oz	100g	Fibre per oz	100g	Protein per oz	100g
Yoghurts										
Natural	15	52	2	6	0	1	0	0	1	5
Apple	23	80	4	14	0	1	0	0	1	5
Apricot	27	95	5	18	0	1	0	0	1	5
Blackcurrant	27	96	5	19	0	1	0	0	1	5
Chocolate	27	94	5	17	0	1	0	0	1	5
Strawberry	25	89	5	17	0	1	0	0	1	5
DESSERTS										
Black Forest gateau	90	319	10	35	5	19	0	1	1	4
Caramel	28	97	5	19	0	1	0	0	1	4
Caramel sauce	87	306	23	80	0	0	0	0	0	0
Chocolate supreme	33	115	5	17	1	5	0	0	1	3
Chocolate sauce	90	318	23	80	0	1	0	0	1	2
Creamed rice	25	88	5	16	0	2	0	0	1	3
Custard powder	100	354	26	92	0	1	0	0	0	1
Delights, made up	40	142	6	20	2	6	0	0	1	3
Jelly cubes	77	268	19	66	0	0	0	0	2	6
Jelly, made with water	17	58	4	14	0	0	0	0	0	0
Jelly, made with milk	25	85	5	15	0	2	0	0	1	3
Milk puddings	37	131	6	20	1	4	0	0	1	4
Mousse chocolate	46	161	6	23	2	7	0	0	2	7
Pancakes	87	307	10	36	5	16	0	1	2	6

FOODS	Calories per		Carbohydrates per		Fat per		Fibre per		Protein per	
	oz	100g	oz	100g	oz	100g	oz	100g	oz	100g
Trifle fruit	43	149	5	18	2	8	0	0	1	2
DRESSINGS (*see also Sauces*)										
Corn oil	255	900	0	0	28	100	0	0	0	0
French salad dressing	139	487	0	0	16	55	0	0	0	0
Garlic mayonnaise	208	734	0	0	23	81	0	0	1	2
Garlic oil dressing	127	443	0	1	14	49	0	0	0	0
Italian oil	126	444	0	1	14	49	0	0	0	0
Mayonnaise	208	734	0	0	23	81	0	0	1	2
Mustard oil	130	450	0	1	15	50	0	0	0	0
Olive oil	251	887	0	0	30	100	0	0	0	0
Salad cream	92	324	5	18	8	28	0	1	1	1
Seafood dressing	92	325	1	5	10	34	0	0	0	0
Soya oil	255	900	0	0	30	100	0	0	0	0
Sunflower oil	255	900	0	0	30	100	0	0	0	0
Tartare sauce	77	271	5	18	6	22	0	0	1	2
Thousand islands	77	273	3	9	7	25	0	0	1	2
Tomato ketchup average	35	123	9	29	0	1	0	0	1	1
Vegetable oil	255	900	0	0	30	100	0	0	0	0
Vinegar	1	4	0	1	0	0	0	0	0	0
DRIED PRODUCTS										
Butter beans	77	273	14	50	0	1	0	0	5	20

FOODS	Calories per oz	100g	Carbohydrates per oz	100g	Fat per oz	100g	Fibre per oz	100g	Protein per oz	100g
Haricot beans	75	270	13	45	1	2	7	25	6	20
Lasagne, egg raw	95	337	21	73	1	2	1	4	3	12
Lentils split	86	304	15	53	0	1	3	12	7	24
Macaroni raw shortcut	94	332	20	72	1	2	1	3	3	11
Pasta bows, shells, twists	94	332	20	75	1	2	1	3	3	11
Pearl barley	102	360	24	84	0	2	2	7	2	8
Peas dried	81	286	14	50	0	1	5	17	6	22
Peas split	88	310	16	57	0	1	3	12	6	22
Rice, flaked, ground, brown etc	100	352	23	81	0	1	1	3	2	7
Spaghetti raw	94	332	20	72	1	2	1	3	3	11
Tapioca, seed pearl	102	359	27	95	0	0	0	0	0	0
FATS										
Beef dripping	252	891	0	0	28	99	0	0	0	0
Butter	210	740	0	0	25	85	0	0	0	0
Lard	252	891	0	0	28	99	0	0	0	0
Margarine	207	730	0	0	25	85	0	0	0	0
Suet butchers block	254	895	0	0	30	100	0	0	0	1
Suet shredded	230	813	3	12	25	85	0	0	0	0
Vegetable oils	255	900	0	0	30	100	0	0	0	0
FISH (*see also Shellfish*)										
Carp	26	92	0	0	1	2	0	0	5	18

FOODS	Calories per oz	Calories per 100g	Carbohydrates per oz	Carbohydrates per 100g	Fat per oz	Fat per 100g	Fibre per oz	Fibre per 100g	Protein per oz	Protein per 100g
Cod fillets	22	78	0	0	0	1	0	0	5	18
Cod fillets in batter	70	244	4	13	5	16	0	0	4	13
Cod fillets in breadcrumbs	61	212	4	14	4	13	0	0	3	11
Coley	28	99	0	0	0	1	0	0	7	23
Dover sole	23	81	0	0	0	1	0	0	5	18
Eel	66	231	0	0	6	19	0	0	4	14
Grey mullet	31	109	0	0	1	4	0	0	5	18
Haddock fillets	22	77	0	0	0	1	0	0	5	18
Haddock fillets in batter	70	244	4	13	5	16	0	0	4	13
Haddock fillets in breadcrumbs	55	191	3	11	3	10	0	0	4	15
Hake	23	79	0	0	0	1	0	0	5	18
Halibut	34	120	0	0	1	5	0	0	5	18
Herrings	66	232	0	0	5	19	0	0	5	17
Herring roe	34	120	0	0	1	2	0	0	7	24
Huss	35	122	0	0	1	5	0	0	6	20
Kippers	61	212	0	0	5	16	0	0	5	17
Lemon sole fillets	23	81	0	0	0	1	0	0	5	18
Mackerel	52	182	0	0	4	12	0	0	5	18
Mackerel smoked	62	218	0	0	4	15	0	0	6	21
Plaice fillets	25	86	0	0	0	2	0	0	5	18
Plaice fillets in breadcrumbs	60	210	5	18	3	10	0	0	4	12
Red mullet	35	122	0	0	1	5	0	0	5	19
Skate	27	94	0	0	0	1	0	0	6	21

FOODS	Calories per		Carbohydrates per		Fat per		Fibre per		Protein per	
	oz	100g	oz	100g	oz	100g	oz	100g	oz	100g
Sprats	40	139	0	0	3	9	0	0	4	15
Squid	23	80	0	0	0	1	0	0	5	17
Swordfish	33	117	0	0	1	4	0	0	5	19
Trout	39	135	0	0	2	7	0	0	5	19
Whiting	22	78	0	0	0	1	0	0	5	18
FISH Frozen										
Cod fillets	24	86	0	0	0	1	0	0	5	19
Cod in batter	69	244	3	10	5	17	0	0	4	15
Cod in breadcrumbs	61	212	4	14	4	13	1	1	3	11
Cod in butter sauce	25	90	1	3	1	4	0	0	3	10
Cod in parsley sauce	23	80	1	2	1	4	0	0	3	10
Cod fish fingers	52	184	5	17	2	8	0	0	3	12
Coley	28	99	0	0	0	1	0	0	7	23
Haddock fillets	29	102	0	0	0	1	0	0	7	23
Hake	23	79	0	0	0	1	0	0	5	18
Lemon sole fillets	23	81	0	0	1	2	0	0	4	16
Plaice fillets	26	91	0	0	1	2	0	0	5	18
Rainbow trout	39	135	0	0	2	7	0	0	5	19
Salmon steaks	52	181	0	0	3	12	0	0	5	18
White fish fillets	23	80	0	0	0	1	0	0	5	18

FOODS	Calories per		Carbohydrates per		Fat per		Fibre per		Protein per	
	oz	100g	oz	100g	oz	100g	oz	100g	oz	100g
FISH Smoked										
Smoked salmon	48	170	0	0	3	10	0	0	6	20
Smoked trout	74	259	0	0	6	22	0	0	5	16
FISH Tinned										
Salmon, pink	40	141	0	0	1	5	0	0	6	20
Salmon, red	44	153	0	0	2	8	0	0	6	20
Sardines in oil	95	334	0	0	8	28	0	0	6	20
Sardines in tomato sauce	51	177	1	1	3	12	0	0	5	18
Tuna in oil	64	227	0	0	5	17	0	0	6	21
FRUIT Fresh										
Apples cooking	9	32	2	8	0	0	1	2	0	0
Apples dessert	14	48	3	12	0	0	1	2	0	1
Apricots	8	28	2	7	0	0	1	2	0	1
Bananas	22	79	5	19	0	0	1	3	0	1
Bilberries	16	56	4	14	0	0	0	0	0	1
Blackberries	8	29	2	6	0	0	2	7	0	1
Blackcurrants	8	28	2	7	0	0	2	9	0	1
Cherries	13	47	3	12	0	0	1	2	0	1
Cranberries	4	15	1	4	0	0	1	4	0	0
Damsons	11	38	3	10	0	0	1	4	0	1
Figs	12	41	3	10	0	0	1	3	0	1

FOODS	Calories per		Carbohydrates per		Fat per		Fibre per		Protein per	
	oz	100g	oz	100g	oz	100g	oz	100g	oz	100g
Gooseberries	5	17	1	3	0	0	1	3	0	1
Grapefruit	6	22	1	5	0	0	0	1	0	1
Grapes, black	14	51	4	13	0	0	0	0	0	1
Grapes, white	18	63	5	16	0	0	0	1	0	1
Greengages	13	47	3	12	0	0	1	3	0	1
Guavas	18	62	3	9	0	1	0	0	0	1
Lemons	4	15	1	3	0	0	1	5	0	1
Limes	10	36	2	6	0	0	0	0	0	1
Medlars	12	42	3	11	1	2	3	10	0	1
Melon, cantaloupe	7	24	2	5	0	0	0	1	0	1
Melon, honeydew	6	21	1	5	0	0	0	1	0	1
Nectarines	14	50	4	12	0	0	1	2	0	1
Oranges	10	35	2	9	0	0	1	2	0	1
Pawpaw	13	45	3	11	0	0	0	0	0	1
Peaches	10	37	3	9	0	0	0	1	0	1
Pears	8	29	2	8	0	0	1	2	0	0
Pineapple	13	46	3	12	0	0	0	1	0	1
Plums	11	38	3	10	0	0	1	2	0	1
Redcurrants	6	21	1	4	0	0	2	8	0	1
Rhubarb	2	6	0	1	0	0	1	2	0	1
Satsumas	10	34	2	8	0	0	1	2	0	1
Strawberries	7	26	2	6	0	0	1	2	0	1
Tangerines	10	34	2	8	0	0	1	2	0	1

FOODS	Calories per		Carbohydrates per		Fat per		Fibre per		Protein per	
	oz	100g	oz	100g	oz	100g	oz	100g	oz	100g
Watermelon	6	21	2	5	0	0	0	1	0	0
Fruit Dried										
Cherries glacé	60	212	16	56	0	0	1	2	0	1
Currants	69	243	18	63	0	0	2	7	0	2
Dates	60	213	16	55	0	0	2	8	1	2
Mixed fruit	71	247	18	64	0	0	2	7	1	2
Prunes	46	161	12	40	0	0	5	16	1	2
Raisins	70	246	18	64	0	0	2	7	0	1
Sultanas	89	312	22	79	0	0	2	7	1	3
Fruit Tinned in Natural Juice										
Apricot halves	13	44	3	11	0	0	0	0	0	1
Fruit salad	14	49	4	13	0	0	0	0	0	0
Grapefruit segments	10	36	3	9	0	0	0	0	0	0
Mandarins	11	37	3	9	0	0	0	0	0	1
Peaches	14	49	3	12	0	0	0	0	0	1
Pears	15	54	4	13	0	0	0	1	0	0
Pineapple	15	52	4	13	0	0	1	1	0	1
Prunes	33	117	9	31	0	0	1	5	0	1
Raspberries	9	33	2	8	0	0	0	2	0	1
Strawberries	10	36	3	9	0	0	0	1	0	1

FOODS

	Calories per		Carbohydrates per		Fat per		Fibre per		Protein per	
	oz	100g	oz	100g	oz	100g	oz	100g	oz	100g
Fruit Tinned in Syrup										
Apricot	20	71	5	18	0	0	0	0	0	1
Blackcurrants	17	60	4	15	0	0	1	3	0	1
Grapefruit	19	68	5	17	0	0	0	0	0	1
Peaches	19	68	5	18	0	0	0	0	0	0
Pears	20	69	5	18	0	0	0	1	0	0
Pineapple cubes	20	69	5	18	0	0	0	0	0	0
Plums	18	64	5	16	0	0	0	0	0	0
Prunes	34	120	9	30	0	0	1	5	0	1
Raspberries	25	88	6	23	0	0	0	2	0	1
Rhubarb	16	56	4	14	0	0	0	2	0	1
Strawberries	21	75	5	19	0	0	0	1	0	1
FRUIT DRINKS *carbonated*										
Cherryade	7	23	2	6	0	0	0	0	0	0
Lemonade, tinned	6	22	2	6	0	0	0	0	0	0
Orangeade	7	23	2	6	0	0	0	0	0	0
Fruit Drinks concentrated										
Blackcurrant squash	82	290	22	76	0	0	0	0	0	0
Lemon squash high juice	42	148	11	39	0	0	0	0	0	0
Lemon, whole	29	103	8	27	0	0	0	0	0	0
Lime juice cordial	27	97	7	25	0	0	0	0	0	0

FOODS	Calories per oz	Calories per 100g	Carbohydrates per oz	Carbohydrates per 100g	Fat per oz	Fat per 100g	Fibre per oz	Fibre per 100g	Protein per oz	Protein per 100g
Orange squash high juice	43	153	11	40	0	0	0	0	0	0
Orange whole	27	95	7	25	0	0	0	0	0	0
Fruit Drinks chilled										
Apple juice	13	45	3	12	0	0	0	0	0	0
Grapefruit juice	11	40	3	10	0	0	0	0	0	1
Lemonade	13	46	3	12	0	0	0	0	0	0
Orange juice	9	30	2	7	0	0	0	0	0	1
Pineapple juice	12	43	3	11	0	0	0	0	0	1
JAM, HONEY & MARMALADE										
Apricot	72	253	19	67	0	0	0	0	0	0
Blackcurrant	72	253	19	67	0	0	0	1	0	0
Bramble jelly	72	253	19	66	0	0	0	1	0	0
Damson	73	254	19	66	0	0	0	0	0	0
Honey average	88	311	23	81	0	0	0	0	0	0
Marmalade average	72	253	19	67	0	0	0	1	0	0
Pineapple	73	254	19	66	0	0	0	0	0	0
Plum	73	254	19	66	0	0	0	0	0	0
Raspberry	74	258	19	67	0	0	0	0	0	1
Strawberry	73	257	19	67	0	0	0	0	0	0

FOODS	Calories per		Carbohydrates per		Fat per		Fibre per		Protein per	
	oz	100g	oz	100g	oz	100g	oz	100g	oz	100g
MEAT										
(see also Poultry & Game)										
Bacon rashers fried										
Back, average	132	465	0	0	12	41	0	0	7	25
Middle, average	135	477	0	0	12	42	0	0	7	24
Streaky, average	141	496	0	0	13	45	0	0	7	23
Bacon rashers grilled										
Back, average	114	405	0	0	10	34	0	0	7	25
Middle, average	118	416	0	0	10	35	0	0	7	25
Streaky, average	120	422	0	0	10	36	0	0	7	25
Beef										
Brisket boiled, average	92	326	0	0	7	24	0	0	8	28
Roast sirloin, average	81	284	0	0	6	21	0	0	7	24
Roast topside, average	61	214	0	0	3	12	0	0	8	27
Rump steak grilled lean	48	168	0	0	2	6	0	0	8	29
Silverside boiled, lean	49	173	0	0	1	5	0	0	9	32
Stewing steak, average	64	220	0	0	3	11	0	0	9	30
Beef corned	61	217	0	0	3	12	0	0	8	25
Beef mince	65	229	0	0	4	15	0	0	7	23
Beef stew	34	119	1	4	2	8	0	0	3	10

FOODS	Calories per		Carbohydrates per		Fat per		Fibre per		Protein per	
	oz	100g	oz	100g	oz	100g	oz	100g	oz	100g
Lamb										
Chops grilled, average	100	355	0	0	8	30	0	0	7	25
Cutlets	105	370	0	0	9	31	0	0	7	23
Roast breast, average	116	410	0	0	11	37	0	0	5	19
Roast leg, average	76	266	0	0	5	18	0	0	7	26
Roast shoulder, average	90	316	0	0	8	26	0	0	6	20
Scrag, stewed	83	292	0	0	6	21	0	0	7	26
Pork										
Chop grilled, average	94	332	0	0	7	25	0	0	8	30
Leg roast average	82	286	0	0	6	20	0	0	8	27
Offal										
Brain calf boiled	40	150	0	0	3	10	0	0	3	12
Brain lamb boiled	35	125	0	0	3	10	0	0	3	12
Heart beef stewed	51	180	0	0	2	6	0	0	9	32
Heart lamb's	33	118	0	0	2	6	0	0	5	17
Kidney lamb's	45	155	0	0	2	6	0	0	7	25
Kidney beef stewed	49	172	0	0	2	8	0	0	7	26
Kidney pig stewed	43	153	0	0	2	6	0	0	7	24
Liver calf fried	73	256	2	7	5	15	0	0	8	27
Liver chicken fried	55	194	1	3	3	12	0	0	6	21
Liver duck	50	176	1	1	2	8	0	0	7	25

FOODS	Calories per		Carbohydrates per		Fat per		Fibre per		Protein per	
	oz	100g	oz	100g	oz	100g	oz	100g	oz	100g
Liver lamb fried	66	232	1	4	4	14	0	0	7	23
Liver pig	53	188	1	4	2	8	0	0	7	26
Liver turkey	48	169	0	1	2	6	0	0	8	27
Oxtail stewed	69	243	0	0	4	13	0	0	9	31
Sweetbread lamb fried	65	230	2	6	4	15	0	0	5	19
Tongue sheep stewed	82	289	0	0	7	24	0	0	5	18
Tripe dressed	17	60	0	0	1	3	0	0	3	9
Tripe stewed	28	100	0	0	1	5	0	0	4	15
NUTS, kernels only										
Almonds	161	565	1	4	15	54	4	15	5	17
Barcelona	181	639	1	5	18	64	3	10	3	11
Brazil	177	619	1	4	18	62	3	9	3	12
Cashew	161	564	6	21	13	46	2	7	5	19
Chestnuts	49	170	10	37	1	3	2	7	1	2
Cob or Hazel	106	375	2	7	10	35	2	6	2	8
Coconut fresh	100	351	1	4	10	36	4	14	1	3
Coconut dessicated	173	604	2	6	18	62	7	24	2	6
Coconut milk	6	21	1	5	0	0	0	0	0	0
Coconut shredded	142	496	9	32	11	40	4	15	1	5
Peanuts fresh and roasted	166	587	3	12	14	49	2	8	7	27
Walnuts	150	525	1	5	15	52	1	5	3	11

FOODS	Calories per		Carbohydrates per		Fat per		Fibre per		Protein per	
	oz	100g	oz	100g	oz	100g	oz	100g	oz	100g
PASTA										
Lasagne egg	95	337	21	73	1	2	1	4	3	12
Macaroni cooked	44	156	10	34	0	1	1	2	2	6
Macaroni raw	94	332	20	72	1	2	1	3	3	11
Ravioli	23	80	4	14	1	2	0	1	1	2
Spaghetti cooked	38	134	8	29	0	0	0	2	2	5
Spaghetti in tomato sauce	17	59	3	12	0	1	0	0	0	2
Spaghetti verdi	37	130	8	29	0	0	0	2	1	4
Tagliatelle	38	134	8	29	0	0	0	2	2	5
Vermicelli	30	104	6	22	0	1	0	1	1	4
PASTES & SPREADS										
Beef paste	64	225	0	1	5	17	0	0	5	16
Beef spread	43	149	1	4	2	8	0	0	5	16
Chicken paste	63	221	1	2	5	17	0	0	5	16
Chicken spread	52	181	1	2	3	11	0	0	5	18
Chicken and ham paste	64	225	1	2	5	16	0	0	5	19
Crab paste	53	186	1	3	3	12	0	0	5	18
Crab spread	38	134	1	5	2	6	0	0	4	14
Salmon spread	40	140	0	1	2	8	0	0	5	17
Salmon and shrimp paste	52	183	1	2	0	0	0	0	5	17
Sandwich spread	58	203	7	26	3	11	0	0	0	2
Sardine and tomato paste	53	185	1	3	3	12	0	0	5	18

FOODS	Calories per		Carbohydrates per		Fat per		Fibre per		Protein per	
	oz	100g	oz	100g	oz	100g	oz	100g	oz	100g
Tuna and mayonnaise paste	67	236	0	1	5	17	0	0	5	17
PATÉS										
Ardennes	99	348	1	4	9	32	0	0	3	12
Breton	90	318	2	6	8	28	0	0	4	13
Brussels	98	345	0	1	9	33	0	0	4	13
Chicken liver	53	186	2	8	3	10	0	0	5	17
Duck and orange	78	274	1	3	7	24	0	0	4	13
Pork liver, mushroom	98	344	2	6	9	32	0	0	3	9
Smoked haddock mousse	78	273	0	1	7	26	0	0	3	11
Smoked salmon	83	292	0	1	7	25	0	0	5	17
Smoked trout	73	259	0	0	6	22	0	0	5	16
Smoked turkey	101	354	0	1	10	35	0	0	3	11
Tuna	108	379	0	0	10	36	0	0	4	15
Vegetable	30	106	2	8	2	5	1	3	2	7
PICKLES										
Beetroot in vinegar	16	57	4	13	0	0	1	3	1	2
Cucumber	8	29	2	7	0	0	0	0	0	1
Gherkins cocktail	3	9	0	2	0	0	0	0	0	1
Mixed pickles	5	19	1	4	0	0	0	0	0	0
Olives cocktail	31	111	1	5	3	10	0	0	0	1
Onions cocktail	3	10	1	2	0	0	0	0	0	1

FOODS	Calories per oz	Calories per 100g	Carbohydrates per oz	Carbohydrates per 100g	Fat per oz	Fat per 100g	Fibre per oz	Fibre per 100g	Protein per oz	Protein per 100g
Piccalilli sweet	24	84	6	21	0	0	0	1	0	1
Red cabbage	6	20	1	4	0	0	1	3	0	2
Sweet pickles	39	136	10	35	0	0	0	0	0	1
PIES										
Apple	51	180	8	28	2	8	1	3	1	2
Cottage	42	148	4	14	2	8	0	0	2	6
Fish	36	128	4	13	2	6	0	0	2	7
Fruit, individual	105	369	16	57	4	16	1	3	1	4
Fruit, pastry top	51	180	8	28	2	8	1	2	1	2
Gooseberry	51	180	8	28	2	8	1	2	1	2
Lemon Meringue	92	323	13	46	4	15	0	1	1	5
Mince	123	435	18	62	6	21	1	3	1	4
Plum	51	180	8	28	2	8	1	2	1	2
Pork Melton	107	376	6	21	8	29	0	0	3	9
Rhubarb	51	180	8	28	2	8	1	2	1	2
Shepherds	35	123	3	11	2	7	0	0	1	5
Steak and kidney	71	250	6	20	4	15	0	0	3	9
PIE FILLINGS										
Apple	18	62	5	16	0	0	0	0	0	0
Apple and blackberry	19	67	5	17	0	0	0	0	1	1
Apple and raspberry	18	62	5	16	0	0	0	0	1	1

FOODS	Calories per		Carbohydrates per		Fat per		Fibre per		Protein per	
	oz	100g	oz	100g	oz	100g	oz	100g	oz	100g
Cherry	27	94	7	24	0	0	0	0	0	1
Gooseberry	20	70	5	18	0	0	0	0	0	0
Strawberry	20	70	5	18	0	0	0	0	0	0
PIZZA										
Cheese and mushroom chilled	76	267	11	40	2	7	0	0	4	13
Cheese and onion frozen	67	233	7	23	4	13	1	1	2	8
Cheese and tomato chilled	75	262	10	36	2	8	0	0	4	13
Cheese and tomato frozen	71	247	7	24	4	13	1	1	3	9
Ham and mushroom chilled	67	234	9	32	2	8	0	0	3	11
Ham and mushroom frozen	65	227	7	24	3	11	1	1	3	9
Tomato, cheese, pineapple and ham	57	198	9	30	2	5	2	2	3	10
Vegetable chilled	63	219	8	28	3	8	0	0	3	9
POULTRY & GAME										
Chicken boiled	52	183	0	0	2	7	0	0	8	29
Chicken roast, no skin	42	148	0	0	2	5	0	0	7	25
Chicken roast, with skin	61	216	0	0	4	14	0	0	7	23
Duck roast, meat only	54	189	0	0	3	10	0	0	7	25
Duck roast, with skin	96	339	0	0	8	29	0	0	6	20
Goose roast	90	319	0	0	6	22	0	0	8	29
Grouse roast	49	173	0	0	2	5	0	0	9	31
Hare stewed or jugged	54	192	0	0	2	8	0	0	9	30

FOODS	Calories per		Carbohydrates per		Fat per		Fibre per		Protein per	
	oz	100g	oz	100g	oz	100g	oz	100g	oz	100g
Partridge roast	60	212	0	0	2	7	0	0	10	37
Pheasant roast	60	213	0	0	3	9	0	0	9	32
Pigeon roast	65	230	0	0	4	13	0	0	8	28
Rabbit stewed	51	179	0	0	2	8	0	0	8	27
Turkey roast breast	29	103	0	0	0	1	0	0	7	23
Turkey roast leg	42	148	0	0	1	4	0	0	8	28
Turkey roast with skin	48	171	0	0	2	7	0	0	8	28
Venison roast	56	198	0	0	2	6	0	0	10	35
PUDDINGS										
Bread and butter	45	159	5	17	2	8	0	0	2	6
Chocolate sponge	100	351	17	58	4	13	1	1	1	5
Christmas	87	304	14	48	3	12	1	2	1	5
Jam sponge	97	341	17	59	3	11	0	0	1	4
Jam suet	90	316	17	57	3	10	0	0	1	3
Rice	43	152	5	19	2	7	0	1	1	5
Sago	39	136	5	18	2	6	0	0	1	4
Semolina	43	151	6	22	1	5	0	0	2	6
Spotted dick	91	320	17	59	3	9	0	0	1	4
Steak and kidney	49	171	3	11	3	10	0	0	3	11
Suet or syrup steamed	92	323	17	59	3	10	0	0	1	3
Tapioca	35	121	5	19	1	4	0	0	2	6

FOODS	Calories per		Carbohydrates per		Fat per		Fibre per		Protein per	
	oz	100g	oz	100g	oz	100g	oz	100g	oz	100g
PULSES & LENTILS *cooked*										
Black eye beans	38	132	7	23	0	0	2	7	3	10
Butter beans	29	103	5	17	0	0	1	5	2	8
Chick peas	44	154	7	24	1	3	1	4	3	10
Green split peas	37	128	6	22	0	1	1	5	3	10
Haricot beans	39	135	6	23	0	1	2	7	3	11
Lentils	31	111	5	17	0	0	1	4	3	10
Mung beans	46	161	8	28	0	0	1	5	4	10
Pinto beans	38	133	6	21	1	2	1	5	3	13
Red kidney beans	29	101	5	17	0	1	3	9	2	8
QUICHES										
Cauliflower	70	246	5	19	5	16	1	2	2	7
Chicken	68	239	6	19	4	15	0	1	3	9
Lorraine	65	230	5	17	4	15	0	0	2	8
Mushroom	73	257	6	20	5	17	0	1	2	8
RICE										
Boiled average	36	127	8	29	0	0	0	1	1	2
Boiled in the bag	96	337	23	81	0	1	1	1	2	7
Curried hot	31	109	7	25	0	1	1	1	1	2
Curried mild	31	107	7	24	0	1	1	1	1	2
Ground, cooked	43	152	7	23	1	5	0	0	1	5

FOODS	Calories per oz	Calories per 100g	Carbohydrates per oz	Carbohydrates per 100g	Fat per oz	Fat per 100g	Fibre per oz	Fibre per 100g	Protein per oz	Protein per 100g
Pudding	43	152	5	19	2	7	0	1	1	5
Pudding tinned creamed	25	88	5	16	0	2	0	0	1	3
SALADS *dressed*										
Coleslaw	34	120	2	7	3	10	1	2	0	1
Coronation chicken	51	179	4	15	3	11	0	0	2	6
Potato	76	266	3	12	7	24	0	0	0	1
Potato with chives	54	190	5	17	4	14	0	1	0	1
Prawn	47	166	2	7	4	13	0	1	1	5
Taramasalata	118	413	2	8	12	41	0	0	1	4
Vegetable	59	208	4	14	5	17	0	2	0	2
SAUCES										
Apple	27	94	7	24	0	0	0	0	0	0
Bolognaise	17	59	2	8	1	3	0	0	1	3
Bread	36	127	5	18	1	4	0	0	1	5
Brown, bottled	32	112	8	27	1	1	0	0	0	1
Cheese	36	127	4	13	2	6	0	0	2	6
Cranberry	39	137	10	36	0	0	0	0	0	0
Curry tinned	15	52	3	10	0	1	0	0	0	1
Fruit bottled	31	107	8	27	0	0	0	0	0	1
Mint	5	18	1	5	0	0	0	0	0	1
Onion	31	110	4	15	1	4	0	0	1	5

FOODS	Calories per oz	Calories per 100g	Carbohydrates per oz	Carbohydrates per 100g	Fat per oz	Fat per 100g	Fibre per oz	Fibre per 100g	Protein per oz	Protein per 100g
Tartare	77	271	5	18	6	22	0	0	1	2
Tomato	24	86	2	8	1	5	1	2	1	2
Tomato ketchup average	35	123	9	29	0	1	0	0	0	1
White savoury	43	151	3	11	3	10	0	0	1	4
Worcestershire	32	112	8	27	0	1	0	0	0	1
SAUSAGES										
Beef fried	76	269	4	15	5	18	0	0	4	13
Beef grilled	75	265	4	15	5	17	0	0	4	13
Chipolatas	81	285	3	10	6	22	0	0	4	13
Cocktail	91	319	4	13	7	25	0	0	4	12
Frankfurters	78	274	1	3	7	25	0	0	3	10
Liver	65	230	2	8	5	17	0	0	4	13
Pork fried	91	317	3	11	7	25	0	0	4	14
Pork grilled	91	318	3	12	7	25	0	0	4	13
Roll, flaky pastry	137	479	9	33	10	36	0	0	2	7
Saveloy	74	262	3	10	6	21	0	0	3	10
SEASONINGS										
Ginger, ground	97	342	18	65	2	6	0	0	3	10
Nutmeg, ground	129	456	8	30	10	35	0	0	2	8
Pepper, black/white	87	308	19	68	2	7	0	0	3	9
Salt, cooking and table	0	0	0	0	0	0	0	0	0	0

FOODS	Calories per		Carbohydrates per		Fat per		Fibre per		Protein per	
	oz	100g	oz	100g	oz	100g	oz	100g	oz	100g
SHELLFISH *meat only*										
Cockles	14	48	0	0	0	0	0	0	3	11
Crab boiled	36	127	0	0	1	5	0	0	6	20
Crab tinned	23	81	0	0	0	1	0	0	5	18
Lobster boiled	34	119	0	0	1	3	0	0	6	22
Mussels boiled	16	56	0	0	1	2	0	0	3	10
Oysters raw	14	51	0	0	0	1	0	0	3	11
Prawns boiled	29	101	0	0	0	1	0	0	6	22
Scampi fried	90	316	8	29	5	18	0	0	3	12
Shrimps boiled	22	77	0	0	0	1	0	0	5	17
Shrimps tinned	27	94	0	0	0	1	0	0	6	21
Whelks fresh or boiled	26	92	0	0	1	2	0	0	5	19
SOFT DRINKS & MIXERS										
Bitter lemon	10	34	3	9	0	0	0	0	0	0
Coca-cola	11	39	3	11	0	0	0	0	0	0
Dry ginger ale	7	24	2	7	0	0	0	0	0	0
Ginger beer	14	49	4	13	0	0	0	0	0	0
Lemonade	6	22	2	6	0	0	0	0	0	0
Lime juice cordial neat	27	97	7	25	0	0	0	0	0	0
Low calorie mixers	0	0	0	0	0	0	0	0	0	0
Soda water	0	0	0	0	0	0	0	0	0	0
Tonic water	8	28	2	8	0	0	0	0	0	0

FOODS	Calories per oz	Calories per 100g	Carbohydrates per oz	Carbohydrates per 100g	Fat per oz	Fat per 100g	Fibre per oz	Fibre per 100g	Protein per oz	Protein per 100g
SOUPS										
Chicken noodle as served	6	20	1	4	0	0	0	0	0	1
Crab bisque	12	41	1	4	0	1	0	0	1	3
Cream of asparagus	16	55	1	4	1	4	0	0	0	1
Cream of celery tinned	15	52	1	4	1	4	0	0	0	1
Cream of chicken tinned	17	61	1	5	1	4	0	0	1	2
Cream of mushroom tinned	15	54	1	5	1	4	0	0	0	1
Cream of tomato tinned	22	77	3	11	1	4	0	0	0	1
Gazpacho tinned	12	43	3	10	0	0	0	0	0	1
Lentil tinned	11	38	2	7	0	0	1	1	1	2
Lobster bisque	18	62	1	5	1	4	0	0	0	2
Minestrone tinned	9	33	2	6	0	1	0	0	0	1
Mulligatawny tinned	11	39	1	5	0	1	0	0	0	1
Onion dried	75	262	16	56	0	1	0	0	3	3
Oxtail tinned	10	36	2	6	0	1	2	6	1	11
Pea and ham tinned	17	60	3	10	0	1	0	0	1	2
Scotch broth tinned	11	40	2	7	0	1	2	2	0	3
Thick vegetable tinned	14	51	3	9	0	1	0	0	1	2
STEWS *cooked*										
Beef	34	119	1	4	2	8	0	0	3	10
Fish	35	124	3	10	2	7	0	0	1	5

FOODS	Calories per oz	Calories per 100g	Carbohydrates per oz	Carbohydrates per 100g	Fat per oz	Fat per 100g	Fibre per oz	Fibre per 100g	Protein per oz	Protein per 100g
STIR FRIES										
Cantonese	40	141	3	9	3	11	1	2	1	2
Chinese	29	102	2	6	2	8	1	2	1	2
Country	28	99	1	5	2	8	1	2	1	2
Oriental	7	26	1	5	0	0	1	5	0	2
Peking	34	119	3	11	2	8	1	4	0	2
Rissotto	21	75	5	16	0	1	1	3	1	3
Southern	16	55	3	10	0	1	1	4	1	3
STUFFINGS *made up*										
Country herb	31	109	6	22	0	1	0	0	1	3
Parsley and thyme	25	86	5	18	0	1	0	0	1	2
Sage and onion	32	112	7	23	0	1	0	0	1	3
VEGETABLES *Fresh* *all boiled except as marked*										
Artichoke globe as served	4	15	1	3	0	0	0	0	0	1
Asparagus	5	18	0	1	0	0	1	2	1	3
Avocado pear raw	64	223	1	2	6	22	1	2	1	4
Beans broad	14	48	2	7	0	1	1	4	1	4
Beans, french	2	7	0	1	0	0	1	3	0	1
Beans, runner	5	19	1	3	0	0	1	3	0	2
Beetroot	13	44	3	10	0	0	1	3	1	2

FOODS	Calories per		Carbohydrates per		Fat per		Fibre per		Protein per	
	oz	100g	oz	100g	oz	100g	oz	100g	oz	100g
Brussels sprouts	5	18	0	2	0	0	0	0	1	3
Cabbage spring	2	7	0	1	0	0	1	2	0	1
Carrots	6	20	1	5	0	0	1	3	0	1
Cauliflower	3	9	0	1	0	0	1	2	0	2
Celery raw	3	10	1	2	0	0	1	2	0	1
Courgettes raw	7	25	1	5	0	0	0	0	0	2
Cucumber raw	3	10	1	2	0	0	0	0	0	1
Endive raw	3	11	0		0	0	1	2	1	2
Kale	9	33	2	6	0	0	0	1	1	2
Leeks	7	24	1	5	0	0	1	4	1	2
Lettuce round, cos, crisp fresh	3	12	0	1	0	0	0	2	0	1
Marrow	2	7	0	1	0	0	1	4	0	0
Mushroom fried	60	210	0	0	6	22	1	4	1	2
Mustard and cress raw	3	10	0	1	0	0	1	3	0	2
Okra raw	5	17	1	2	0	0	0	1	1	2
Onions raw	7	23	1	5	0	0	1	5	0	1
Onions fried	99	345	3	10	10	33	1	9	1	2
Parsley raw	6	21	0	0	0	0	3	0	1	5
Parsnips	24	86	5	18	0	1	0	5	1	2
Peas	15	52	2	8	0	0	1	2	1	5
Pepper [chilli] raw	11	40	3	9	0	0	1	1	0	1
Pepper red or green raw	4	15	1	2	0	0	0	0	0	1
Potatoes new	22	77	5	18	0	0	1	2	0	2

FOODS	Calories per		Carbohydrates per		Fat per		Fibre per		Protein per	
	oz	100g	oz	100g	oz	100g	oz	100g	oz	100g
Potatoes old baked	31	107	7	25	0	0	1	3	1	3
Potatoes old	23	80	6	20	0	0	0	1	0	2
Pumpkin	6	21	1	5	0	0	0	1	0	1
Radish raw	4	15	1	3	0	0	0	1	0	1
Salsify	5	18	1	3	0	0	0	0	1	2
Shallot raw	14	48	3	10	0	0	0	0	1	2
Spinach	9	30	0	1	0	1	2	6	1	5
Spring greens	3	12	0	1	0	0	1	4	0	2
Spring onion	10	35	2	9	0	0	1	3	0	1
Swede	5	18	1	4	0	0	1	3	0	1
Sweetcorn	35	124	7	23	1	2	1	5	1	4
Tomato raw	4	14	1	3	0	0	0	2	0	1
Tomato fried	20	69	1	3	2	6	1	3	0	1
Turnip	4	14	1	2	0	1	1	2	0	1
Watercress raw	4	14	0	1	0	0	1	3	1	3
Yam	34	119	9	30	0	0	1	4	0	2
Vegetables Frozen										
Beansprouts	9	33	1	5	0	0	0	1	1	3
Breaded courgettes	81	283	10	36	4	14	0	0	1	5
Broad beans	14	48	2	7	0	1	1	4	1	4
Brocolli spears	9	32	1	5	0	0	0	0	1	3
Brussels sprouts	6	20	1	2	0	0	1	3	1	3

FOODS	Calories per		Carbohydrates per		Fat per		Fibre per		Protein per	
	oz	100g	oz	100g	oz	100g	oz	100g	oz	100g
Cabbage	6	21	1	4	0	0	1	3	0	1
Carrots	7	24	2	6	0	0	1	3	0	1
Carrots, baby	6	20	1	4	0	0	1	3	0	1
Cauliflower florets	3	10	0	1	0	0	1	2	0	2
Corn on the cob	35	124	7	23	1	2	1	5	1	4
Corn cobs, baby	8	28	1	3	0	0	1	5	1	3
Courgettes sliced	5	16	1	4	0	0	0	0	0	1
Green beans	2	8	0	1	0	0	1	3	0	1
Mushrooms	4	13	0	0	0	0	1	3	1	2
Peas	14	48	2	6	0	1	3	12	2	6
Peppers, mixed	5	16	1	2	0	0	0	0	0	1
Ratatouille	13	45	2	6	2	2	0	0	1	2
Spinach chopped	7	26	0	1	0	0	2	6	1	5
Vegetables Tinned										
Beans baked	18	64	3	10	0	1	2	7	1	5
Beans broad	14	50	2	6	0	1	1	5	2	6
Beans butter	17	59	3	9	0	0	1	5	2	6
Beans curried	29	101	6	21	1	3	2	7	1	5
Beans green whole	10	36	2	7	0	1	1	2	1	2
Beans kidney red	29	101	5	17	0	0	3	9	2	8
Carrots	5	19	1	4	0	1	1	4	0	1
Mushrooms	4	13	0	0	0	1	1	3	1	2

FOODS	Calories per		Carbohydrates per		Fat per		Fibre per		Protein per	
	oz	100g	oz	100g	oz	100g	oz	100g	oz	100g
Peas garden	13	47	2	7	0	0	2	6	1	5
Peas marrowfat	23	80	4	14	0	0	2	8	2	6
Peas petit pois	23	82	5	16	0	0	1	3	1	5
Peas processed	23	80	4	14	0	0	2	8	2	6
Potato Jersey	15	53	4	13	1	3	1	3	0	1
Ratatouille	13	46	1	4	1	3	0	1	0	1
Sweetcorn	21	75	5	16	0	0	2	6	1	3
Tomato	5	16	1	3	0	0	0	0	0	1
VINEGAR										
Cider	1	3	0	1	0	0	0	0	0	0
Distilled	1	4	0	1	0	0	0	0	0	0
Malt	1	4	0	1	0	0	0	0	0	0

Section 3

Alcohol listings

Alcoholic Drinks	Calories per	
	100 ml	pint
BEER		
Best bitter	32	180
Brown ale	28	160
Guinness	37	210
Pale ale	32	180
Lager average	29	165
Lager german	40	225
Stout bottled	37	210
Stout strong bottled	39	220
Strong ale	72	405
Yorkshire bitter	42	235
CIDER		
Dry	36	203
Medium	43	242
Sweet	42	236
Strong	35	297
Vintage	101	568

	Calories per		
	100 ml	¹⁄₆ gill	glass
SPIRITS			
Brandy	220	55	
Gin	220	55	
Tequila	205	52	
Vodka	220	55	
Whisky	220	55	
WINE			
Red	70		75
Rose	80		85
White, dry	70		75
White, medium	75		85
White, sweet	95		100
Champagne	75		85
Sherry, dry	110		125
Sherry, medium	75		85
Sherry, sweet	95		100

OTHER USEFUL TITLES

The Handbag Hip and Thigh Programme 95p
A commonsense low fat approach to slimming. This programme not only helps you shift unwanted fat but also ensures you maintain your new shape with delicious recipes and menus. All you need to know for a beautiful body.

The Handbag Fat and Calorie Counter 95p
An easy to use fat and calorie counter. The listings of the fat content of foods will help you to identify which ones to each and which ones to avoid.

The Handbag Weight and See 95p
The weight loss game that makes slimming fun. Contains the calorie values of over 1000 different foods as well as a chart to encourage and record your progress.

The Handbag Beat Cellulite 95p
With this book you really can beat cellulite. It explains exactly what cellulite is, how to recognise it, what causes it and how to cure it.

The Handbag Hip and Thigh Exercises 95p
Easy and practical exercises for problem areas. Really clear illustrations will guide the reader through these effective exercises for toning the hips and thighs.

The Handbag Low Fat Meals 95p
Delicious new low fat recipes. With excess fat now recognised as a major contributor to killer heart disease, this book is definitely a must for every family.

The Handbag Count your Calories 75p
A revised enlarged and updated edition with values in calories per ounce and metric, listing more than 1000 foodstuffs commonly in use. This proven and hardy best seller has now sold more than 5 million copies.

The Children that Time Forgot £4.99
These true case histories deal with children's memories of *former* lives on earth. They reveal clues to a pre birth dimension of time and space.

Available from bookshops & newsagents or send payment and stamped addressed envelope direct to Kenneth Mason Publications Ltd, Dudley House, 12 North Street, Emsworth, Hants PO10 7DQ .
Telephone 0243 377977.